The Charm of Making

The Creation of Merlin

&

The Secret of The Grail

Kennan Taylor, MD

A catalogue record for this book is available from the National Library of Australia

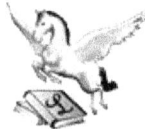

Linellen Press
265 Boomerang Road
Oldbury, Western Australia
www.linellenpress.com.au

Contents

"I must create a system, or be enslaved by another man's. I will not reason and compare: my business is to create."

William Blake, *Jerusalem*

Preface

This work can easily fall between stools. There are potential social, psychological and religious conclusions that can be drawn from it, but any such approaches have been employed in this account to embellish other viewpoints that are being explored and presented. Nor has it been drawn into some of the intellectual themes that present themselves, such as the significance of history to the present, or a comparative study of the symbolism inherent. I have also not been seduced into a theory of dreams, although one could readily be drawn from the account.

Instead, this narrative is to place all these fields, and the unanswered questions they raise, into a personal and revelatory narrative that I refer to loosely as 'soul-making'. In a world relatively devoid of meaning and direction, as reflected in the poverty of our belief-systems, attitudes and values, as well as the becalming effect of climate-change, war, poverty and recurrent pestilence, I have attempted to go to the core of the narcissistic and isolated outcome of this void and, somewhat ironically, illustrate that, with enough sincerity, a spiritual outcome is attainable through such a core inquiry. Not only this, but also such an attitude is necessary, even essential for the revitalisation of a western culture that lacks depth and connection to a transcendent basis of individual existence.

I have drawn on Merlin, and later Perceval, as mythic personnel in tradition, but also as core spiritual identities. These figures have a literary, but not necessarily a literal representation – if a strictly historical Merlin is being sought, disappointment will ensue. Merlin is discovered within ourselves and here I am providing some of my own psychological mapping. This is not to negate the central Christian figure of Jesus, but to put both he and that Tradition into context, and see figures – like Merlin – who straddle the real-mythic boundary, are capable of revitalising our spiritual languor in the West. With this, I also see that they need to connect to the core of our individuality, talk to our souls and our creative expression in social and community settings.

To do this, it is essential that we look to the literature and traditions espoused herein as mature and still alive. By mature, I mean that we do not arrogantly see them as somehow more primitive than our current modern position; in fact, I contend the reverse may well be the case. I would also add that seeing myth in modernity as untrue or even dishonest is a strange inversion, bordering on the demonic in its literalisation of a foundational truth of our existence.

This is a narrative that is easy to criticise, particularly with the self-exposure it contains. The degree such judgement can be suspended is the degree to which it may talk to the reader, my literary skills notwithstanding. Yet a central thesis is that Merlin is archetypal and lives within our culture still, and some of us more distinctly than others at the individual level. Similarly with the Grail, which I contend has no distinct historical representation, but talks to us nonetheless, revealing the secrets of our life's journey, meaning and purpose.

Orientation

I am approaching this work somewhat differently to others I have written. Although the third and last of a series of narrative works derived from my life experiences, the former two were written in a post hoc kind of manner; that is, recounting life experiences and my conclusions about them. By way of contrast, this work will evolve somewhat differently. It continues the theme by being based unapologetically on such personal life experiences, but I have allowed the ideas to flow in as I write, with parallel research and the evolution of conclusions that have and still do surprise me. Having started, I did not know where this work would end, because – and I suspect was also the case with the writers of the film *Excalibur* – I had presumed that it would be entirely about Merlin, but this is clearly not what eventuated. So, I have let the content intention drop and just followed the flow and, if I dare say it, responded to a kind of spiritual imperative.

What has surprised me is that the Jungian orientation that started this journey and which, from a professional stance I eschewed many years ago, has emerged as a framework that vaguely underpins the inquiry. It has confirmed to me that some of Jung's thought I found difficult in my professional days I still find problematic, although most of his insights I still stand by, particularly those of his more mature years.

In brief, this work could be seen as a quest that individuation best describes and which Merlin and the Grail Quest provide the context for. And the concept I have most wrestled with is that of the self, the orientation that has guided me beyond the personal and other related content. (Henceforth, I will differentiate Jung's more transpersonal concept of the self from the day-to-day reality one of the more personal 'self' by italicising the former). Yet it is psychospiritual disciplines such as alchemy that have substantially informed me and which preoccupied Jung's later research. Dreams, dreaming and dreamwork have been and still are staples. This is not a Jungian treatise however. Rather it is my own work ... ideas, concepts and all. I believe that is what individuation is all about and Blake endorses "I must create a system or be enslaved by another man's". The fact that the conclusions of my maturity once again often align with Jung's has been a quiet but rewarding fulfilment.

Within the framework of my own life journey, I have taken existing ideas and explored them further. Having watched *Excalibur* countless times, this has led to reading and research that has both surprised and excited me. Beyond the more popular ones, the books I have on the Grail had remained comparatively unexplored. In contrast, I have quarried Merlin in some detail prior. The result of this is that Part One held few in the way of surprises – the general direction and outcome was not a fantastic departure from what I had already concluded. I just needed to put it into some sort of order around my own life experiences.

In contrast, Part Two has been a revelation. I rather suspect there are more surprises to come but, rather as in one way of appreciating the journey of Perceval and his various namesakes, I am learning patience.

Writing Approach

This work is fundamentally imaginative and creative; it will not be footnoted or referenced. This is not an academic work, and I have also not read much of the medieval source material directly, except when in the body of other works. I incline to modern writers as diverse as the English-Russian Nikolai Tolstoy, the Scottish RJ Stewart, and the French Jean Markale with their poetic dispositions, speculative ideas, creative approaches and lashings of intuition. Unlike the scholars, I rate intuition of a higher order than mental cognition, which has defined too much of the argument surrounding Merlin and the Grail to date. These and other writers may be referred to in the account itself, with their and other relevant books I have used listed at the end. In this manner, the reader will be able to follow my flow relatively uninterrupted, then extend their reading to others inspired by anything I write and refer to.

I have a strong academic, intellectual and scientific background. Yet, I eschewed this in favour of a practical medical career. I then followed my passion, initially inspired by Jung, and pursued my own heritage and ancestry whilst living in Australia. Ultimately, these pursuits and other life circumstances led me here, to Merlin. In the maturity of my years, I have chosen to devote time and practical research to him, because I have found his story to parallel my own in so many ways. But this does not surprise me nor make me unique, as I know he is talking to many. I will be bringing my own story into this account when appropriate, often frequently, and I trust significantly. In this way, I hope to make Merlin's story one of our era, to assist in lifting us out of the moral darkness that eclipses us in the early 21st Century. Maybe this is why Merlin is returning.

Yet Merlin's story inevitably, it seems, could not be isolated and left without recourse to the Grail legends. Reluctantly initially, and prodded by *Excalibur's* manner of dealing with the Grail, I started to look at my dreams more deeply and dusted off the relevant works in my library to launch into Part Two. Then I found myself immersed in a further adventure, one which has not ceased even with the completion of this account. Expect loose ends.

Beyond this, there is no particular structure or order to this work. The framework, referred to a little earlier, just about encompasses it all. As we delve deeper into the territory, other avenues and paths will open up for exploration. My style is somewhat journalistic and based on a career of many thousands of hours of "talking therapy" with patients and clients; the rub-off from this will inevitably influence my writing, as it does all forms of instruction and presentation I undertake. I hope it inspires you and – excuse the phraseology – talks to your heart. If so, then I, or Merlin, has done his job and weaved his magic.

Original Dream

I had the following dream over forty years ago, at a time when my life was starting to unravel and I sought therapeutic assistance. My fledgling medical career was at a significant juncture and I had also commenced an intense love affair that indirectly ended my marriage. A series of apparent coincidences led me to a Jungian analyst; my therapeutic adventure had begun. I am sharing the dream below, with the ensuing and more recent associations and connections.

I have looked at this dream every which way since I had it. This was initially from a Jungian perspective: It was the first dream of my therapeutic analysis, and is often referred to as the *Original Dream* of such an analysis, hence the name of this section. Such a dream is considered important, in that it may define not only the analytic direction, but also one's life more generally. As in Jung's concept of *Individuation*, it is fatalistic, in the authentic meaning of that word – my preference is the Old English term for fate or destiny, being *wyrd*.

Over the years I have teased out the personal elements, as well as taken alternative perspectives to look at it, most notably that of alchemy. I can relate the dream with its elements and symbols to other significant dreams with similar archetypal themes; but the intention now is to look at it specifically from a more spiritual, alchemical and mythic perspective, most particularly with Merlin and the Grail themes.

As the dream is read, let the images resonate in the imagination and allow any associations that emerge. I have given you mine below, immediately after the dream; but remember, they are mine, and not for endorsement or agreement. Instead, I would like the salient images and any associations to them to stand on their own authority, as I follow the personal and collective threads into the spiritual, mythic and other perspectives outlined earlier.

> *I am looking at the sea from high above, as if on a map; it's the Pacific Ocean. A new island is emerging; it is called Hiroshima. It is a city island and I am now in the city square surrounded by old and gracious buildings. In the centre is a fountain. The sculpted centrepiece is like an organ-pipe cut off at the top. As I gaze at it and look, almost seeing through it, it becomes a vast octagonal jewel.*
>
> *I'm now in the countryside of the island working as a doctor. Julie, my receptionist, takes the patients' cards from the cupboard. There are two; the 'original' man and woman. I have seen the woman before, but not the man, although I have treated his son. The man enters, emerging from a mist. He wears a jacket and white polo-neck sweater; he is worn out, exhausted. I look in the cupboard where there is a jar, I realise I may need to use a vice to open it.*
>
> *(Original Dream of Analysis, 1978)*

The creation and/or destruction theme, or creation:destruction, is readily apparent in the initial setting. (NB. I use a colon with no spacing here, and generally as in the more familiar *mind:body*, as a way of reconciling opposites, so effecting some sort of unification that is not – as yet – present in our Modern English language or, indeed, our routine mental frameworks.) Peace:war is implied in the names Pacific and Hiroshima; the latter place name is also putting the dream into a more contemporary context. This complex of issues is compounded by symbolic features of birth, and a sexual background is implied. Also present are the material elements of fire and water, and the concept of power. The primal and sexual background has, in the past, not been highlighted. It is present nonetheless; it permeates the dream, along with birth, death … and later resurrection.

Then I become personally immersed in the dream, possibly implying my own birth which the emerging island would reinforce, as well as my new 'birth' in Australia after emigrating from England. To my mind, the island indirectly resonates with the mythical Lemuria by its mythical location, and indirectly with the fabled Atlantis. The *city square* has personal associations to the old city of Stockholm, being the site of personal sexual discoveries during my explorative youth. Maybe somewhat significantly because of this location, Hyperborea has not been previously noted in any detail, although it feels present now. The square also resonates with my alma mater of Oxford University, but even more so with Saint Bartholomew's Hospital, where I later trained as a medical doctor. Tradition, learning, healing and medicine are features that could be drawn from this complex of associations, depending on the context.

The fountain infers water, although it is not actually seen or flowing here. It is placed at the centre of the featured icon, which I imagine to be stone. There is an alchemical and Grail-like positioning and reference in this, as with the 'jewel in the stone' – stone and jewel are both Grail symbols – although the implied stone of the fountain also has a more metallic look and feel. Yet somehow this is beyond the more masculine phallic and sexual images in the *sculpted… cut off organ pipe* embedded in the feminine, with the implied flow of water, as well as the potential birth-like aspect of the jewel emerging from the stone. In addition to amniotic or other sexual fluids, semen is a loose association to any flow, if the phallic reference is considered. Does the *cut off* refer to castration, I now wonder; not just in the Freudian context, but as the wounding of the Grail or Fisher King, in Part Two. Viewed in reverse: The Grail radiates out through the feminine to the masculine, before manifesting within tradition, learning etc. as a quadrated manifestation.

The Grail image itself is associated more directly with stone (sculpture), water and then jewel. It seems to manifest from either beyond the primal imagery or in an alternative state of consciousness, or even both; rather like the *original man* I will come to in due course. The jewel is doubly quadrated and even Celtic as a potential *medicine wheel* image, colour (maybe green), and is also – presumably – valuable. As a stone it may be an emerald, reinforcing the generally Celtic and, more specifically, Irish associations. I recall now that Ireland is an island, rather like Australia. This makes me wonder whether there are pre-historical inferences in the island, such as in the Lemurian, Hyperborean and other associated myths hinted at earlier.

The second half of the dream begins with a paradox: It is originally a city island in the first part of the dream, although I am now in the country. Indeed, over time and in reality I have returned from the city to the country, both as doctor and also to live. This was not at all on my agenda at the time of this dream. Julie (not her real name), who was my actual receptionist at the time, reinforces the rural aspect and my heritage, being a West Country Girl from England with a broad local accent. While there are some erotic associations with Julie, these are not significant in the dream, or my knowing of her (no pun intended).

Elsewhere, I have previously noted the significance of the original man, woman and son from a religious and personal family perspective, even to giving them a Freudian and oedipal interpretation. But what does the term *original* mean? It is somewhat vexing (as with *vice*, to which I will come) and could imply something more primal with Garden of Eden implications, or be more archetypal and alchemical. It does reinforce that this is an 'original' dream, in the analytic context. There are no clear avenues extending from all this, presently. In the dream I have seen and hence treated medically the mother and son, although I have not seen the father, who is now the main focus of attention.

The Celtic theme is reinforced in the triadic structure of father-mother-son, which is simultaneously religious with its Trinitarian association. The connection with the first half of the dream, where it is from the masculine perspective through the feminine that the Grail is 'realised' is mirrored here, and is also compatible with the order in the actual Grail legends. This is a distinct pattern in the legends, where the Grail seeker asks the question and heals the wounded King through the ritual of the Grail, as revealed and displayed by the feminine. It should be noted here that I do not ask some rather obvious questions of or about the man at this time.

But I am not the son; I am the doctor, the healer, and I am seemingly there to treat the father. He emerges from the – possibly Celtic – mist and, again, as from another reality or dimension like the jewel. So, he is a representative of the Grail as its wounded guardian, the Fisher King. His garb is modern, which is a surprise, but then so is Hiroshima. He is also quite English, being personal and smartly traditional. He is tired and worn out, as the Fisher King is in the Grail legends, which puts me in a Perceval role, as well as being the Druid-healer. Maybe the Fisher King's wounding being sexual is of further significance? (These associations will become apparent.)

I am vexed by the jar and needing a vice to open it, the contents of which are relatively obscure' although by inference it is possibly involved in the man's healing. There are lots of word associations that can be applied to the word *vice*, particularly around sex and power, but I am left dissatisfied with these; there feels to be more. At present, the alchemical association of the jar as an alchemical *athanor*, or healing vessel, and hence a resonance with the stone-jewel, seems to fit best. This implies an elixir of life, if considered healing with respect to the father's ailments. The vice clearly indicates I will need strength or power to access this and hence heal him.

There the dream ends. I don't open the jar, possibly a metaphor: I don't ask the right question? The dream is then left hanging. I have made a couple of further connections, such as the symbolic otherworldly location from which both the jewel and the man emerge, and the triadic nature of the dream, but have reached no substantive conclusions: I do not expect this dream – or any other – to directly do this, that is my task. I am also in the role of healer and, indirectly maybe, Grail seeker. There is little direct evidence of Merlin's presence.

The healing is in the realms of sex and power, which is an inevitable conclusion to draw. Vice also implies the nefarious side of sexuality, and is where any power is actively engaged. This is a question within myself that I have not yet fully answered and is one of the intents in this account. Power is also present with Hiroshima (nuclear power), as well as elemental fire. Sex:power as a dyad is something to ponder further now. But now, with all these loose threads left up in the air, I will move on.

The dream has a subtle chronological movement from spirit to soul in the two halves: It is as if spirit is manifesting and directing the dreamer, or informing his soul. This is a common pattern in mystical literature, when the timeless realms interpenetrate our consensus reality; one could see the movement of the Old to the New Testament in this light, for example. Yet spirit and soul together permeate the whole dream. In *Excalibur*, the movement is reversed: The personal realms, in which Merlin has a significant influence, then move to the more collective, transpersonal or spiritual realms of the Grail Quest, where his influence is less involved and more transcendent.

This latter pattern will be more adopted in this work as Parts One and Two respectively, with Merlin as my guide. Yet the interpenetration of the two realms should not be segregated by such an outline; they are prominent in both the film *Excalibur* and the dream, as well as other dreams and material to come. It may be better to envisage this pattern as circular in two dimensions and spiral in three, where the timeless realm interpenetrates temporal reality by flowing in and out, backward and forward, encompassing deep themes such as birth and death in acts of creation … and as indicated in the actual *Charm of Making* itself. Consider the whole work as a tapestry, where the various levels are woven together to form an overall creative pattern.

There are, other dreams that I intend to introduce into this work, two significantly. The first of these follows in Part one, the second extends from the Original Dream above and is in Part Two. This first one is the final occurrence of a recurring dream that I had in my childhood. I am unsure of the time period of this: I was, at the time, quite relieved for its disappearance. But after I began analysis, it re-emerged and kept beckoning me to explore it further. What will follow in due course is this dream, a summation of what I now appreciate about it, and how it connects to the Original Dream, specifically the second half. In this process, I hope to introduce Merlin so that he can, indirectly maybe, undertake the navigation of Part One hereon.

PART ONE

The Creation of Merlin

Introduction

To a varied extent, I have lived with most, if not all of the features that have been and are still ascribed to the assumed person that we know as Merlin. In this, I know I am far from alone. This has been a progressive process of realisation, a psychic birthing of something or someone that has lasted my whole life. Now, in these later years, I am coming to see him as myself emerging from the mists of eternity, as I give him form in this time and place … if this does not sound overly pretentious, paradoxical or enigmatic … a conjunction of soul and spirit, if you will; concepts themselves that will be frequently visited, elucidated and revisioned in this work.

As with the *Charm of Making*, immortalised in John Boorman and Rospo Pallenberg's epic 1981 film *Excalibur* – a purported rendering of Malory's 15thC classic prose work *Morte d'Arthur* – life is being created and breathed into the present era by the alchemical dragon of existence through the portal of death and life. The actual *Charm of Making* is given here with a Celtic pronunciation, as its sources are apparently from the Gaelic language group:

> *Anall Nathrach,*
> *Urthvas Bethud,*
> *Dochiel Dienve.*

Or in Old Irish text, as this is the most likely origin of the screenwriters oral version:

Anál nathrach,
orth' bháis's bethad,
do chél dénmha

Although it is one of many variations, the interpretation generally favoured is:

Dragon's breath,
the charm of death and life,
thy omen of making.

Serpent is a frequently used alternative to Dragon; I favour the latter, particularly as it features in word and image frequently within the movie itself. Although both have elemental associations, *dragon* is particularly associated with the element of fire, lacking with *serpent*; a feature also highlighted in the movie. Sometimes *spell* is used instead of *charm* in line 2, without the initial *the*, as well as *charm* for *omen* in line 3, without *thy*. The differences here are subtle and their usage may boil down to personal preference, which may also indicate a lack of knowledge and appreciation of such subtlety and depth in the modern mentality, including my own.

Come hither ye ancestors
Emerge from the mists
Let life be created

This is an alternative translation and rendering of the *Charm of Making*. It is now a generation since it came to light and I now do not recall how I chanced upon it, except it was offered in the exchanges I was involved in around the *Charm* with its origins and meaning, which I was engaged in online at that time. I suspect that, given some of the resonances with the Original

Dream, it was my joint rendering from a variety of interpretations provided by a Gaelic scholar I was dialoguing with. This may personalise the content, but does not invalidate it.

This particular rendering connects with the dream via the *mists*, which also reinforces the Celtic flavour. The original man could then be seen in the context of an *ancestor* and that the dream itself may be a creation charm, as indicated in some of the associations to the jar containing the *elixir of life* amongst other alternatives. It may also be relevant to see the mists as representing a marginal or liminal space connecting the known and the unknown in an act of creation.

With this rendering, I am establishing a connection between my personal material and the more impersonal realms of translation, meaning and the like that are present in the *Charm*. Because I may have had a hand in this particular translation, a lack of validity could be posited, or the creative act those many years ago could portend what I am working here with now. I would add this may not be at variance with the creation of the *Charm* by the creators of *Excalibur*.

Surrounded by obfuscation and enigma, the Charm's origins and sources have not been revealed by the author(s). Although in the past I have been involved with others in trying to trace these origins, it is not my preference henceforth. Instead, my intention is to use it as a kind of *leitmotif* throughout this work, as a magical spell leading to a deeper appreciation of both Merlin and his role, if any, in the Grail Quest.

I have often felt Merlin within me, although I have usually not recognised him as such … or maybe I have denied him. It is a relatively easy thing to avoid the archetypal patterns of existence, instead favouring one's personal narrative, although the latter is somehow included in the former. Such denial can feel comforting, yet sometimes irresponsible: It is not without psychological or physical danger if such patterns beckon strongly, as any shaman would attest and psychiatrist judge. Merlin nearly died several times … so have I. And with each grim reaper sortie, I began to realise him more, which may belie the deeper significance of such events. But did Merlin ultimately die or, like Arthur, pass to another realm of existence?

At a deep level, Merlin magically arranged the circumstances of Arthur's birth, as well as creating himself within the world, as in the charm. Yet somewhere in this process is the flaw that led to the round table broken asunder, Camelot's disintegration, and the confederation of knights dispersed in their apparently hopeless search for the Grail. Or maybe this flaw was a necessity for the Grail Quest that issued forth from the calamities, then and still now? Shamanic resonances, again. We may still be seeking an Arthur in our present time of need, but more deeply and spiritually we thirst for Merlin. In modern guise he pops up as a Gandalf, Dr Who or Harry Potter, as well as in the seemingly endless variations provided in science fiction and fantasy literature. Having been created, he is far from dead, and he certainly is not buried.

I have misgivings about Merlin's apparent rendering as Gandalf in JRR Tolkien's *The Lord of the Rings*. It seems a close match and is thus attractive in modernity, but *The Lord of the Rings* is more in the lineage of a Grail legend continuation where traditionally Merlin's input is minimal, if present at all. Its deep and rich mythological content is put into a more Biblical framework, with a strong Gnostic flavour, and Tolkien's own views of religion, sexuality and the feminine cast a shadow over a work that was designed to rehabilitate or even create an English mythic and spiritual heritage.

I see *The Lord of the Rings* as a rearguard action of the Christian tradition within Tolkien himself, attempting in so many ways to integrate and rehabilitate the Mage that is Merlin, but within his own worldview. This is, of course, quite acceptable and in the tradition of the Grail that it be so revisioned to meet the demands of the Age. With Wagner's operatic *Ring* cycle, *The Lord of the Rings* provides a broad and detailed perspective that has much to offer modernity, even if only by contrast. However, I find *Excalibur* and its continuation more in the Grail legend tradition, and through its creative imagery a readily available and significant comment on Merlin and his role in the present, as well as the prophetic future.

Is this why the Grail remains elusively out of our grasp, unreconciled by incomplete or inadequate Christian solutions? Gandalf is too wise and his shadow projected elsewhere. Yet, more than this, he has an idealised, distant, and sanitised view of sexuality and the feminine. As a somewhat asexual figure, he does not resolve any of the enigmas that his medieval predecessor left to posterity. Rather, there are many features of Gandalf that resonate with Merlin's ongoing presence in the various written continuations of the Grail legends, originating in the late 12thC. Tolkien's work is brilliant as a modern rendering of archetypal and mythic material; however, he remains a Christian apologetic, and this is one flaw in the Grail legends that I want to engage.

But is the grave Merlin's final destination? Because he is not dead … or is he? All the films and literature say not … maybe: Yet another link to Arthur's enigmatic demise. So, Merlin remains still one step away from our grasp. One reason for this is that we have lost a great secret; we have not asked the core question: What exactly is magic? Whilst Merlin is a prophet, healer and counsellor, does this make him a magician? What magical acts did he actually perform? Then there are the further questions that emerge from these, such as the nature of death, the role of the feminine, and much more.

This one great question of the nature of magic is what I have sought to address in my own life, though not always aware that this is what I was doing. It is reflected here in this account, and ultimately why I wrote it. Because, in so addressing it, I have paradoxically found Merlin. And Merlin lives within me. Yet there is more to this story, as the medieval writers recognised: There is the connection to the Grail, and Merlin's role in the Quest. The two are intimately connected in a way that I believe these medieval writers tried to, but did not ultimately answer. So keen were they to use this material for the advancement of Christianity that the story lost its roots in the Pagan Traditions that preceded it … and which have re-emerged in our time.

Merlin is the connecting figure in these unanswered questions. But to accept the challenge and approach answers to these questions I believe that psychic patterns, such as the personal *shadow*, as in Jung's terminology, must be examined through the agencies of power and sexuality. With what emerges from such an elucidation is the levels of the personal and the collective, and how they resonate and harmonise with each other; because traditions that include disciplines such as shamanism, magic and alchemy, can restore a magico-mythical perspective. Finally, it will be seen how this process gives depth and a purposeful outlook on the challenges of our time, and addresses the fundamental need of re-establishing a psychospiritual solution to them.

Whilst Merlin walks through the entire territory expressed here, he will be more prominent in the first of this two-part work. *Excalibur* is similarly structured; although my offering is not plagiarism or a simple coincidence. It is because Merlin's emergence and journey best demonstrates some of the more personal issues I raise and encapsulate in the above paragraph. But the Grail story is more collective by its very nature and will best address the latter two points of that paragraph from a more objective position. The voice in the first part that is more distinctly 'mine' may then move to one that is more feminine in nature: The reasons for this will be apparent in the telling of this in Part Two.

Introducing Merlin

Merlin, as a name known to us through the works of Geoffrey of Monmouth whose creation he is, is based on several figures from history and legend. In this respect, he is more substantial than Arthur, who is largely a product of the later medieval period after the Norman conquest.

Prior to Geoffrey, a mythic identity in the 5th and a more substantial historical one in the 6th centuries seem to largely define Geoffrey's creation, although it is the earlier, more legendary figure who has been built on in the ensuing Arthuriad. Yet the 6thC version contains more significance for me and material that is relevant to this account. For this reason, as I build on the figure of Merlin, I will be paying detailed attention to the book of Geoffrey's in which he is portrayed, which carries many differences to his earlier mythic incarnation that is more popularly appreciated in modernity.

However, in spite of Geoffrey's apparent failure to bring these two differing pictures of his Merlin into some sort of unity, I believe it is potentially done if the more human picture of the 6thC version is given voice, even if it would appear, rather like it would with Arthur, to diminish the rather glorified version of the popular imagination. This more humanistic position is, I maintain essential, if Merlin and his entourage are to be less rarefied and 'talk' to us today.

Merlin has become sanitised to the point that even his less than pure actions, such as the magical engineering of Arthur's birth, are understood in some sort of greater, purer and more spiritual perspective, which then leaves his dark side – his *shadow*

– elsewhere. Yet he does have one, and it is seen in the 6thC version of the Mage in a more personal manner, and becomes available to us in a psychological sense. In this context, I see Geoffrey's attempt at unification as quite valid and appropriate, which is why I wish to restore the balance in this account. Otherwise, his shadow side is left to others, most notably the figure of Faust, whose more individual challenges in his quest for meaning have left that side of the human personality rendered dark, in a way that approximates his doppelgänger, Mephistopheles. Magic is thus left with a bad name.

Ironically, in the earlier mythic version of Merlin in the 5thC, there is a figure called Faustus (the latinised version of Faust), who wrestles with the individual path to spiritual realisation by championing the approach of the Celtic priest, Pelagius, and who leads a religiously pure life. Of further interest is that this Faustus is the son of Vortigern, by a nefarious union that mirrors the birth stories of both Merlin and Arthur. I will come to Vortigern, who represents a very fluid axis around which the events of the 5thC appear to satellite. But the detail of this, and the further story of the contending visions of magic that Merlin and Faust represent, must remain unstated here; they will form a future work.

So, to Geoffrey and his Merlin, and the detailed account of the 6thC version that will form the basis of much that will follow, including the Grail.

Merlin's Background

There now seems little doubt that the figure of Merlin, as described in Geoffrey of Monmouth's mid-12th century book, *Vita Merlini*, is a vaguely historical figure of the late 6thC. He lived in the rural and forest borderlands of the Scottish Lowlands with their Irish, Northern Welsh, and North of England connections. Here he is rather identified with the name of *Myrddin*, although this is one name amongst several. This Merlin in the *Vita* contrasts with a man of the same name in his earlier work, *The Prophecies of Merlin,* that became embedded in Geoffrey's other notable and more literally successful book, *The History of the Kings of Britain.* This Merlin would have lived in the late 5thC and therefore seemingly a different figure, although there is no clear historical record of him.

This latter figure of Merlin in the earlier penned *Prophecies* is more prophetic, mythical and even archetypal than the rustic, mad and shamanistic figure in Geoffrey's later *Vita.* The former are the characteristics of the 'Merlin' that exist in early Welsh myth and legend as Myrddin, and was maybe Geoffrey's source for his Merlin. Actually, Geoffrey latinised Merlin as Merlinus Ambrosius, being Myrddin Emrys in Welsh; Ambrosius being a connection to Nennius, to whom I shall come. In the *Prophecies* Merlin is located more southerly in South Wales and the English West Country regions, and he is also now a prophetic youth. These various works of Geoffrey's were written between 1130 and 1150 in Oxford, reputedly a significant Druid site of yore, as well as being where I went to university.

Regarding Merlin, *Prophecies* was written first in 1135, and the one that led Geoffrey on a meandering path via the *History* into the remaining more anthological material that comprised the significantly later *Vita.* However, both history and tradition imply that he would have known of Myrddin, at least in fable, particularly at the time of writing *Vita.* Given the differences between the two works, it is of interest to me that he should use the name Merlin in both. He also claimed an unknown source for his description of the prophet, a not unusual thing; the 9thC clerical figure of Nennius would fit the bill, but it could equally well imply an intrapsychic authority. One other notable feature of this earlier Merlin, in the *History* that contains *The Prophecies*, is his association with Arthur, significantly like Nennius.

Effectively, Merlin begins his story into the present with Geoffrey. Like Nennius before him, Geoffrey was a religious man, but with distinct Celtic affinities and associations, specifically Welsh. This reinforces the close yet somewhat parallel nature of these traditional Pagan influences to the Christian Church at this time, whereas with the subsequent written material – particularly the Grail legends – there is an attempt to incorporate such influences more into mainstream Christianity. Unlike Arthur, references to a character resembling Merlin in the first millennium are relatively detailed, even if often only implied or indirect in legend, as with Myrddin maybe and others I will come to.

Confusingly and by way of contrast, to date the sole written reference to Arthur appears to be his involvement in the Battle of Camlann in 537 CE, where both he and Mordred succumbed, although Arthur may have been whisked away to Avalon for healing and rebirth, according to legend. Interestingly to me, this reference provides a feasible connection between Arthur at that time, and the more historical material surrounding Vortigern and the Anglo-Saxons later in the 5thC, as described by Nennius. Negating this is the fact that Gildas, a Church historian who lived from 500 – 570 CE makes no mention of Arthur, but does mention the Battle of Badon around the turn of the 6thC in which Arthur supposedly fought, as referenced by Nennius in his 9thC account named as the *Historia Brittonum*. Also, and somewhat paradoxically and confusingly, *Vita* contains an account of Arthur's journey to Avalon: Was this deliberate on Geoffrey's part, to either confuse or connect the apparent two Merlins?

Indeed, the actual name of Merlin arises only with Geoffrey; why it was adopted is surrounded with conjecture, but I dismiss relatively the overly simplistic explanation that it was to avoid association of *Myrddin* with the French *merde*, or shit, he was already named Merlin in the earlier *History* after all. There have been some academic and research attempts to connect Geoffrey's Merlin in the *History/Prophecies* with the Myrddin of the latter 6thC in the *Vita*, particularly through some further linguistic gymnastics around his name. I find these unsatisfactory. The time discrepancies also mitigate against the association becoming a unification, although there are some intriguing psychological and mythical possibilities that I will come to that indicate how the two Merlins resonate with each other. Maybe it is for these or other reasons Geoffrey wrote of both as one person, because it seems obvious to me that he did, otherwise I find no clear and plausible reason for the Merlin figure in the *Vita* and the one in the *Prophecies* to be connected by name, as on the surface they present as quite different people. Maybe Geoffrey sees them as unified in an archetypal manner.

Geoffrey, somewhat enigmatically, made only vague attempts to conflate these two figures; as personalities, they seem relatively easily dissembled. I see this desire for unification as a product of our modern mentality, in its search for order and rationality, and tried by many in tackling these apparent problems. The rational unification process remains unresolved and in my opinion inevitably so for reasons that will emerge in this work, such as with the points raised in the preceding paragraph. Maybe in Geoffrey's mind such rational unification was unnecessary. The two figures reflected aspects, levels, reflections, or even psychic *harmonics* of the same figure and possibly served different functions. I contend that disciplines such as depth psychology and alchemy provide a better framework within which to see this process.

Interestingly, given Merlin's Pagan background and nefarious parentage – he was considered by Geoffrey to be the son of an incubus, specifically the Devil in the Christianisation process, and a mortal woman – he gained momentum in his more mythic form and became increasingly identified with Arthur and later the Grail legends during the subsequent medieval period from Geoffrey's time on. However, I contend that the resonances with the shamanistic Myrddin of later in the 6thC are important to understanding Merlin more holistically, as well as to connect him with his Celtic background and Pagan Tradition more generally. Was this also Geoffrey's intention in writing *Vita*?

There is much modern reference to the various themes of Merlin's apparent predecessor(s), in spirit, if not in name. These explorations flow temporally not just backward historically, but also forward from the depths of pre-history. They exist more in the mythic sensibility and narrative of oral tradition, and have clear shamanic undercurrents. Various stories can be traced that emerged from this oral tradition into written format. The formal written material prior to Geoffrey largely resides with church writers, such as with the Welsh monk Nennius in the early 9thC. In Nennius' *Historia Brittonum* Merlin is called Ambrose, sometimes referred to in the Welsh as Emrys, and is located in the late 5thC with the supposedly tyrannical warlord Vortigern. Here he is simply a fatherless child and recounts the story of the dragons; there is prophecy, but no magic. My impression is that this material bolsters the Romano-British position around the kings that included Arthur vis-à-vis the Saxon or other threat. This Ambrose even features in the regal lineages and may even have been a king in Wales. Geoffrey directly links Ambrose with his Merlin rather than more mythic Welsh figures; I find this significant.

Christianity overlaps the whole story, particularly the documented material, making the prior oral material of tradition of interest to my sensibilities. For several hundred years after Britain was exposed to Christianity there was a distinct branch, the Celtic Church, which provided a continuum of sorts with the prior Pagan traditions. Indeed, much of the Celtic Druid tradition would have easily fitted into the Celtic Church in these subsequent early centuries of the new millennium, probably seamlessly. Even the clerical Geoffrey, with his Welsh background, had such leanings as late as the 12thC. In spite of the Synod of Whitby in 664 CE, which saw the Roman version become the Christian mainstream in Britain, I contend that the Celtic version flowed as an undercurrent, then and even into the present. This undercurrent intrigues me and is a major background theme of this present inquiry.

Henceforth, I will follow Geoffrey and refer to our figure of myth and history as Merlin, in spite of there being no direct record of such a named person prior to his books. He is now immortalised with this name, and is the way we recognise him in modernity. One reason for this acknowledgement is that, as one goes back in time, personal names were less common and significant; titles and various impersonal descriptions were more commonly used. Merlin could have been a title, for example, as this was not uncommon as a kind of description, such as *The Merlin*. It could also have been a reference to his trade as a shamanic and magical figure. It may, intriguingly, refer to nobility. I say all this, because the various alternative names of the enigmatic Mage have suffered a similar fate in this historical pursuit; they can lead to becoming lost in confusion by taking this wrong path into the forest, viewing it with a modern sensibility alone.

However, some loose ends may need identifying before I move on. I suspect there are more immediate religious and political motives to Geoffrey's accounts than have been fully acknowledged. Nennius' earlier prophetic picture of Ambrose-Merlin is considerably elaborated by Geoffrey, even to introducing clear magical acts, although these may be considered more the manipulation of natural forces, including his engineering of Arthur's conception and with supposed building of Stonehenge; the latter being an impossibility in the given time frame. Rather like Nostradamus' prophetic material in his *Quatrains*, we have yet to exhaust the relationship of the *Prophecies* to the turbulent local events of Geoffrey's time, including his own social and political position.

The desire to have Arthur in one's regal lineage is similar to earlier Kings wanting the shamanic and semi-mythical Pagan god Woden in their genealogy. This was certainly the case with Henry II, who succeeded Geoffrey's contemporary, Stephen, with his attempt to have Arthur – and Guinevere – seen as interred in English and Christian soil at Glastonbury Abbey. These are intense psychic forces and their manipulation is not only an act of power, but approaches magic; were both Nennius and Geoffrey involved in such acts? I suspect so.

Unfortunately, the deeper we go into this material from a research and academic perspective, the more obscure things seem to become. This is why I am trying to reverse the way we look at it; from the inside out, so to speak, giving primacy and authority to mythic and narrative material, prior to interpreting it historically and factually. It is fundamentally the way this work is directed.

Themes

Beyond the central theme of magic, there are also various other complementary and overlapping ones that demand consideration. Merlin is often portrayed as a *Druid*. However, the Druids as a priestly ruling class were eradicated in the mid-first century CE at the same time of Boudicca's independence revolt;

both were simultaneously and ruthlessly dealt with by the colonising Roman legions. Given its antiquity and status in Celtic Tradition, Druidry would have survived with an underground existence after these traumatic events, maybe in the less confronting Bardic tradition and subsequently within the emerging Christian Church, which was of a more Celtic persuasion prior to the Roman Church exerting her influence. Alternatively, it may have existed and even flourished – and exist still – in the shamanic realms beneath or beyond the reach of the immediate Roman or later Church authority.

However, there is no direct association of Merlin with Druidry, except in the modern imagination fed over the last millennium by various writings from Geoffrey onward, and more particularly in the last few centuries with its waves of Druid revivalism. Instead, other associations are emphasised with him, such as prophecy and magic. However, the Pagan sources provide ample material of various figures who make up much of the narrative material of Merlin's life, and here history and myth merge into a more archetypal framework. Jungian thought will assist in this reframing process.

I will be looking in a more intuitive manner at the pre-Roman period, as well as within the subsequent pre-Christian period, being from the time of Jesus until Rome formally adopted Christianity with Constantine's conversion in 312 CE. It must be noted that this 4thC transition was not sudden, but represented a progressive trend. It was not until later in the first millennium that Britain became more formally Christianised and the stories around Merlin and his various synonyms are embedded in these religious fluxes, including the Anglo-Saxon and later Viking polytheistic worldviews. The Church effectively succeeded in colonising Britain in a sustained manner religiously, where the Romans did not militarily; I see both as political and with strong influences on any written history.

The archetypal picture of the prophetic Ambrose-Merlin in the late 5thC is the one that has been consolidated and built on, rather than the more historical figure of Myrddin-Merlin in the later 6thC, espoused by Geoffrey in *Vita*. The flow of time can be viewed and examined in its chronological orientation from the beginnings of history to the present, to capture these broader themes and their significance. But historical and anthropological methods are both retrospective and also tend to be reductive, being defined by the attitudes and values of our modern culture rather than those of the time in question; that is, they can miss what isn't being looked for. By way of contrast, authentic reconstruction may rely on mental functions that may fly in the face of science and rationality, but I believe it can be both a complementary and also more holistic way of examining the past, and specifically the figure of Merlin.

In passing, it must be remembered that there were other significant influences in the period between the Romans' departure from Britain (early 400s CE), which had already spawned the introduction and emerging religious dominance of Christianity, and the period prior to Geoffrey's books (1130 - 1150). These include the Anglo-Saxon migrations so significant with Arthur's story, as well as the later Viking ones. The former exist in Merlin's account in the earlier 5thC story, specifically with respect to Arthur. But I believe the later and more Scandinavian or Viking input has been minimised or excluded, yet is relevant to our modern understanding. I consider the overlapping Germanic and Scandinavian mythic influences, most specifically the figure of Odin, or Woden as he is known in Britain, to be greatly underestimated.

Woden, the shamanic, mythic, and sometimes godlike figure of mainly Anglo-Saxon Pagan tradition, overlaps not only Merlin, but also the Jesus story. The Merlin of the *Vita* is quite shamanic and Wodenesque in my opinion, making his written inclusion in the overall narrative interesting, particularly from a man of the church. This similarity to the life of Jesus may well be a factor in how Merlin was viewed in the medieval period and his inclusion in some of the Grail legends. An added theme is the northern rune material that, for centuries, rivalled the Roman script in usage throughout the first millennium; its significance has not been included, and I will address this lack. Alchemy and some other esoteric developments are also underestimated in importance, although they are embedded in the early prophetic story of Merlin, which I will be elucidating and further exploring.

As stated, consideration should be given to the circumstances in which Geoffrey wrote. It was a turbulent period following the suppressive Norman conquest in 1066. It was also politically unstable in Britain at the time Geoffrey wrote his books in the 1130 – 1150 period; Stephen was king until Henry II assumed the throne as the first Plantagenet king in 1154. The period was particularly troubled with Stephen's reign being interrupted by the claims to the throne of Henry's mother, Matilda. These events would have had a significant effect on his writing, and hence how Geoffrey saw Merlin, as well as some of his intention in the character he conveyed publicly: I suspect more than a little duplicity here.

All this notwithstanding, Geoffrey's *History* work, inclusive of Merlin's *Prophecies*, was enormously popular; it was a veritable bestseller of the time. It also spawned other copies, similar works, and anticipated a larger continental output that progressed to the Grail legends. So, it was seminal, and a catalyst to many cultural themes of the time. How much it's success was a consequence of contemporary events, as well as Geoffrey's own preferences and role in them, is maybe difficult to gauge, but they appear significant to me. It was also Henry who began the search for Arthur's grave that resulted in its apparent but erroneous discovery – conveniently with that of Guinevere – in

Glastonbury Abbey later in the 12thC. This certainly would have suited the foreign Plantagenet claim to the throne and its lineage, as well as the Church's appropriation of Arthur in a Christian context. It also indirectly preserved the Welsh and Celtic interests, at the expense of their more Northern Germanic cousins.

The significance of the *History* in the emergence of the Arthurian and Grail legends is well recognised; although the latter would be a relative distraction, was I to pursue these legends too far along the exclusively Christian route. Instead, I am interested that medieval writers saw fit to continue with Merlin's presence, when it might have been easier to leave him at Arthur's birth, which is where Geoffrey, following Nennius, did in his writing. I will be extracting various themes from this body of material, specifically the Grail itself, but also the role and place of the feminine, sexuality, and specific others, such as ritual and magic. As others have done, and like I am doing with Merlin himself, these themes need properly restoring to their pre-Christian and Pagan roots, and differentiated from the religious and political influences of the period, particularly if they are to be reconstructed in modernity with authenticity and a voice to the future.

However, I want to continue with an open spiritual attitude and not be drawn too much into a Christian apologia for this later medieval period, particularly and inevitably as consideration of Merlin leads us indirectly and sometimes, somewhat paradoxically, directly to the Grail. Instead, I favour a landmark 15thC work *Le Morte d'Arthur* of Thomas Malory, like Boorman and Pallenberg in *Excalibur*, as a kind of closure to this medieval portrayal of this erstwhile prophet and magician, although I will not be exploring Malory directly. Other tools of interest include alchemy and, to a lesser extent, astrology; in fact, they are probably more than mere tools, because I believe they define our understanding of Merlin better than any other framework, particularly the Christian one; astrology, in particular, permeates the *Prophecies* in considerable detail, although I will not be exploring the content of them in this work. I will also be using medicine, specifically mental health; psychology, specifically Jung; and occasionally other modern disciplines, to both enrich and further this examination.

Framework

It is of great interest to me that many modern writers often associate human qualities that describe something psychologically significant in configurations of four. Jung would love this: He saw the number four to be a core archetypal pattern of consciousness or the transpersonal *self*, analogous to the four directions; human temperaments (choleric, melancholic, sanguine and phlegmatic); the esoteric elements of tradition (earth, water, air and fire); and even in his own typology (thinking, feeling, sensation and intuition). As a tangential example, a modern psychiatrist, Irwin Yalom, describes the core human anxieties or fears to arise from isolation, death, freedom (think about that one) and meaninglessness. This pattern may stem from Aristotle's *causes* (formal, efficient, material and final); although maybe more interestingly and relevant is Socrates' supposed qualities that make up madness or ecstasy being the erotic, prophetic, artistic, and healing, which have a distinctly shamanistic flavour.

Now we are getting closer to Merlin. Norma Goodrich describes him as a priest, teacher, healer, and astronomer. John Matthews sees him as a shaman, prophet/seer, magician, and sage; then he seems to ruin the pattern by adding a fifth, the lover: Well, possibly not, maybe this is a sexual, alchemical and relationship portal into equivalent feminine functions. To this we will return, because I find the lover to be a significant, relatively undervalued, and sometimes trivially dismissed aspect of Merlin. Instead, she is commonly portrayed in other female figures and images, somewhat distant from the Mage himself. Seeing the feminine in Merlin's inner landscape may be a significant factor in his modernisation, and also his future; a future as being psycho-spiritually driven and creatively constructed, including within this account.

To start with shamanism: Is Merlin a shaman? I will follow Stephen Glosecki's view of shamanism, so as not to get caught in the anthropological or cultural arguments about its origins, and who is – or isn't – entitled to call him or herself a shaman. This is simply because Glosecki, a scholar of OldEnglish, puts shamanism in a creative and archetypal framework that transcends such cultural divisions. Shamanism is basically an animistic spiritual worldview and tradition, which works with the concepts of ensoulment and metaphysical power. Merlin is certainly this, but what about the specific functions of the shaman?

Again, following Glosecki, there are four qualities to consider. The shaman leads a marginal or liminal existence, an undervalued concept that will be restored in modern and ritualistic significance in this work. He or she works with ecstasy, where ecstasy is seen as trance-like states or altered states of consciousness. Mircea Eliade, the modern anthropological founder of shamanism as a discipline for exploration, defines the shaman as "a technician of ecstasy". The shaman becomes such by a process of initiation, often through severe illness and madness. The art of healing, and the use of specific tools, both physical and metaphysical, round off Glosecki's four. Note there is no direct reference to magic, prophecy, or power in this definition, which someone like a Carlos Castaneda would incline to. Such metaphysical functions do not register as easily on the anthropological radar, it appears; interestingly though, they do resonate with Socrates' directly and with Glosecki's more indirectly.

As an aside: It may seem that I have focussed excessively on the number four, when others like three might have equal significance. Am I being too Jungian? A little further clarification might help. Simply put, four is quadrated and a pattern that is fixed and static, it appeals to our modern mental sensibility. Three is less solid, more fluid, and indicates dynamic process over static pattern, as in past-present-future, or even Hegel's abstract philosophical triad of thesis-antithesis-synthesis. I will have more to say about three – which is thoroughly Celtic – when we move to more abstract and metaphysical concepts like magic, prophecy and power.

These various functions are present in the radiating extensions of Goodrich and Matthews, as described earlier. This pattern is also present in the Old English concept of *Wyrd*, or fate, which is defined as destiny, as well as embracing magic, prophecy, and power. They – the interlocking features – are all there in various groupings described in the preceding paragraphs, if you care to look. The term *power* will also occur repeatedly: Power is indispensable to magic, and is both poorly understood and also denigrated by psychologically regressive trivialisation in our largely materialistic culture.

Personally, I believe that magic itself is not one of these stated qualities, but something more distinct: It is spiritually supervening, or metaphorically and alchemically distilled from the others, as constituents or elemental qualities. Like power, I don't think magic can be defined or qualified in this simplistic and materialistic way. And, in fact, the story of Merlin – whichever one you use – makes little reference to clearly defined magical acts as our modern sensibilities would see or understand them; instead, prophecy is more supreme and power is also accentuated. The relationship of power to magic is enigmatic and intriguing, explaining as it does the success of modern writers such as Carlos Castaneda and Starhawk.

I also believe, as I have hinted toward already, that alchemy is vastly underestimated in the Merlin story, particularly as a magical discipline. Magic, as considered by the modern mentality, says more about our misunderstanding of the physical and metaphysical realms, and their inter-relationship, than it does about the formal esoteric discipline of magic itself. I trust this will be better revealed and understood as we progress.

Recurring Childhood Dream

I get off the noisy school bus and begin the walk up the driveway to the farmhouse of our family farm, which is out of sight from the road over a rise. I am alone and it becomes silent and seemingly darker as I start walking. From across the open field a large black shape appears on the horizon, it looks like one of the electricity pylons that traverse the farm elsewhere, but here feels animated and showing an interest in me. Although it does nothing but appear and be directed toward me, I am frightened that I won't get home.

When it appears on the last occasion I have the dream, I determine that I have the capacity (within the dream) to awake any time I want. I will not have the dream again, seemingly as a consequence of this choice, although I do not recall exercising it in the dream.

(Recurring Dream of Childhood, late 1950s)

Although the feeling of being on the school bus was convivial in the dream, I generally recall it being tedious, unenjoyable and sometimes with overt physical bullying of me. The only time I stood up to the driver for his personal behaviour or attitude toward me, regarding an event that was occurring on one such trip; my father took the driver's self-protective position after he asked why I had walked home from the neighbouring village, after I had been ejected from the bus. I also recall that my parents took little interest in any bullying, as it was somehow "part of growing up."

I mention these preliminary points for two reasons. Firstly, the reversal from trauma to the conviviality presented in the dream may represent a loss of innocence produced by this trauma. It also was the expulsion from this innocence that seemed to lead to an apparently deeper trauma: Or did it? Was the deeper trauma a symbolic representation of something that stood behind the bullying? I may have believed so at the time, now I think somewhat differently. The second is my father's decision in supporting the driver's account of what happened over mine, his son. I felt bereft, mistrusted and isolated; there was a similar loss of innocence in my view of my father with what I experienced as betrayal.

In the winter period, it was usually dark when the half-kilometre trek home began. My sister, some sixteen months younger than I, usually accompanied me. The relatively short period between our births is a brief window into the lack of nurturing that I experienced in those early years. My explanation of my sister's absence in the dream is that during this period she was often in hospital or otherwise absent as a result of a farm accident when she was five, which resulted in her losing more than half of her left hand. The much later discovered complicity of my parents in this trauma might explain and compound my sense of isolation and aloneness.

In essence, my relatively young, and maybe ill-suited, parents brought significant sexual and birth trauma to their marriage. In many ways, my coming into the world two years after a traumatic pregnancy loss represented an attempt to heal this. Yet I was still a kind of replacement to that significant loss in these prior events; I was not *seen* as myself, but as *another*. Behind this interpretation stands the deeper concept of the *changeling*. The original Celtic concept is that there is an exchange of babies where one from the *faery realm* is substituted for a human infant. In my case, this experience is extended over time. With Christian interpretations, a changeling is often seen as demonic, deformed or imbecilic. When we come to see Merlin's parental background, there are some remarkable similarities.

Then after my sister's birth, my father conducted a long-term affair that stood significantly as a backdrop to the farm accident, when my sister was caught in the psychic crossfire between all three adults involved. I remained relatively innocent of and oblivious to all this illicit sexual background, although my sister knew and was attracted to the drama. I escaped to the fields, animals and the *home* that I would find there. Boarding school at age thirteen was the final escape: I never returned to the family home to live permanently.

This is the background that I can now convey relatively dispassionately. It is hardly unusual or severe in comparison to others, particularly my sister. However, in the rather prosaic way things can be discussed in modernity I guess that, unlike my sister, my wounds did not show. Instead, it was the collective nature of the environment, land, and the creatures that occupied it that sustained and nurtured me. It would be tempting to see the pylon-shape in this context as a symbol of the trauma threat and that my desire to escape it (*I determine that I have the capacity… to awake any time I want*) shows a strength and maybe psychic maturity. However, why then would the dream haunt me after I began analysis twenty years later? Maybe the apparent capacity to escape was somewhat repressive, even if necessarily so at the time for survival reasons.

Although animated, the pylon did not directly threaten me, but I responded with fear, as if it had. I was concerned I could not then get home; something of an irony. I also discovered much later that the direction it merged from was a field on the edge of the farm where my father would meet his lover. So, it came from a background of early childhood and probably generational trauma that could be a ready and more accurate explanation of subsequent events in my life. It is not that I contend that personal trauma is not significant, but that such trauma is more of a window into deeper issues that maybe the pylon is portraying here. It is not an either-or, it is a both-and phenomenon.

These personal events and patterns are in and of themselves enough to explain the dream and its effects, if a more reductive and quasi-Freudian approach is taken. But the image of the pylon begs further appreciation. Although one was present as a typical skeletal metallic structure on the farm, this was neither its location nor where it was coming from. Also, the figure is dark and full, with the resultant shape being more like an arrow or barb, which pylons can sometimes appear as. Yet I have wondered whether the actual barbed upper section is not a disguised or capped head, but shoulders, such that the figure has been decapitated.

The shape is not unlike the *Tyr* – ↑ – rune of Nordic mythology, a point of personal interest to me, because I have developed an active interest in the runes, particularly of the Old English or Anglo-Saxon variety. Tyr is a mythic god who loses a hand in a sacrificial manner in dealing with primal forces; sacrifice is a significant feature in my life and also the legends of the Grail. My sister lost half her hand. Runes are also used for divination and hence have a prophetic quality; divination is associated with magicians and shamans of all cultures.

From childhood, certain images or concepts have had a lingering or frightening effect on me. Seeing an early production of Charles Dickens' *Tale of Two Cities* on television, with the guillotine descending onto a supposed figure below the image and offscreen, chilled me and still does in a way that other forms of execution do not. The guillotine is not unlike the pylon in image. Decapitation is a significant feature in Celtic myth. My mother also recalled how the concept of the *Ice Queen* would terrify me, although I do not recall this. I have recently wondered whether these issues represent a connection to the Faery land of Celtic lore.

A pylon is a conveyor of electricity, rendering the image distinctly energetic, although not threatening in and of itself. It relates to sexuality, via my father's activities, so the sex:power complex is present. It will be recalled in the Original Dream that the fountain was somewhat metallic with phallic features that stood in front of the more feminine features I elucidated. It seems that all of these features can be connected to the fountain image of the Original Dream and I now consider them in some sort of continuum, dragging with them the traumatic features of my personal narrative, but pointing to a deeper level of a more transpersonal nature. Whereas as a child I found the pylon frightening, I now wonder whether he/it was "calling me home". It is time to link some of these features to Merlin.

After writing the above, I recalled an experimental hypnosis session I undertook about a generation ago, with a very skilled and gifted clinical hypnotist. Effectively, I went into a hypnotic or liminal space and there underwent a visionary experience of the dream, where I was back on the driveway and looking at the pylon advancing over the horizon. I walked toward it and merged into its huge frame. I then continued to walk toward the farmhouse. When I got there, I found the buildings to be older, more rustic and wooden, and aflame. I walked around the building, realising it would be burned to the ground. People in unfamiliar dress were watching, but there was little they could do. I did not know how the blaze had started, but it did not seem to be related to the dismayed people around it.

Sometime afterward, I made the mental connection with a

neighbouring village called Monks Kirby, or church (kirk) of the monks. I realised that somehow the responsibility lay here, and that the old farmhouse I lived in had been built on a Pagan site. Somehow, this all made sense to me; not only of the visionary experience, but also of some childhood ones, such as the Druid figure that I will come to. Following this session, I had two further spontaneous visionary experiences:

I have images of a monastery on the burned site and monks around, but it is now a more recent site. In a shed area is a grave and in it is a druid-like figure with an emblem, possibly a triquetra, around his neck. He has been executed. I experience him as being a priest whom the Romans had taken to the nearby spinney and crucified on a tree, having first torn his eyes out. There is a sort of past-life connection with him. I see him in a priestly role in a circle somewhere at the end of the drive, with many men standing around in a circle and dancing (this preceded the crucifixion).

On another occasion, I am in the field from whence the pylon used to emerge. It is as if I am watching a man, who may also be me, as he is executed by beheading with an axe or sword. I later wonder whether his throat is cut, maybe as well, at the same time. Prior to this had been a sense of a feminine element to the figure, maybe around Boudicca, distinct blond hair. I have an affinity with this man, an ancestor. Again, there is something of a 'past-life' feeling. His death may have been a sacrifice, the beheading may be to take his knowledge and wisdom – or conversely preserve it, Celtic-style. Was he killed by assailants, or his own people, the head to be used for veneration? I recall the pylon figure, headless, and my childhood fear of the guillotine. Was the burning in the hypnotic session done by assailants, or his own people?

Am I dealing here with the early Anglo-Saxon period post-Roman occupation, with the village Monks Kirby's proximity and potential religious significance, or Boudicca's earlier time?

I offer these experiences not as an explanation of the dream, or indeed anything that ensues from it and related further in this account. Indeed, by the end of this account, they may well still be unexplained and relatively unintegrated. To me they imaginatively embellish the dream and other childhood experiences, adding psychic information to the mix. They are not a kind of indirect way of bringing in past-life or so-called karmic experiences into the account, nor any implied belief in them and reincarnation. I reserve my opinion about such explanations of psychic experience, instead trusting the creative imagination process that is leading me more deeply into a psychic world that can only be minimised or belittled by such manoeuvres and cognitive explanations, which only inevitably reduce and rationalise.

What was also strange was that the land I had recently brought here in Australia, and the buildings I had erected over a generation ago and some time prior to the hypnotic session, bore a strange yet distinct resemblance to the farm and immediate surrounds, even down to the natural geography. Whilst this may not be surprising, the fact that I had not made any such connections to this time, my time at my present home was. I had done all this subliminally, as an act of recreation; was it simply reductive in meaning, an attempt to recreate my childhood? And why would I do that? I did not see that period with great happiness or any fondness: So, what was I trying to create? Maybe it had more to do with the future?

I have little to add to these experiences presently, although they raise the issue of heredity, ancestry, and memory of other lives. I had not recalled these two visionary deaths, although the beheading and crucifixion motifs are strong for me and occur at various points in this account.

Forgetting and Remembering

I will start with a personal story, being my first encounter with Merlin. To do this, I will focus on the intrapsychic experience of visions and memory, as I did with dreams earlier, rather than the mental one of information and explanations from the outer world. This may appear scattered and somewhat random: The psychic world is fluid and variable; it speaks in symbol and metaphor, association and analogy, not fact and history. It is bound neither by space nor time in the way we are accustomed to see it in our daily reality. It is appreciated more artistically, more than a science; a picture that is being created, rather than a factual or cognitive document of accepted and acceptable data. It demands a leap of faith, making the psychic world of the soul the main fulcrum around which the figure of Merlin will constellate, giving the spiritual dimensions an opportunity to talk to a listening recipient.

I don't actually remember this as a distinct childhood memory, as in the recall of a clear remembered prior event, but it nonetheless feels like one, and also seems more substantial the older I get: An old Druid lived in the garden. Not specifically at the bottom of it though, because there wasn't really a bottom. And he feels more like a misty presence now than a specific memory, or even a series of memories, as if the mists now seem to enshroud him. The lawn stretched sideways following the long farm house frontage and he lived in one further corner, in clear view of and close to my upstairs bedroom window. Here the flat lawn gave way to a rise and a large tree stood in the corner. He lived near there on the rise, maybe in a recess or hut. But I don't recall him as an imaginary figure in my childhood, also he was not created by me. I often used to climb that tree, and the thought that a Druid lived underneath never occurred to me as a child when around or up that tree during the day.

I do recall a more specific memory: A vision of seeing myself as a psychoanalyst one day. It was in a neighbouring area of the farm and was an isolated experience; it was of me becoming or being a psychoanalyst and it only happened once, as I recall. Unlike the Druid, it actually was me. An older greyer version maybe, but definitely me. The Druid seemed as other, or another, but not me. Well, not then, now I don't know. The psychoanalyst seemed like a portal into an unknown future, whereas the Druid did not, so I have assumed – rightly or wrongly – a window into a more distant past beyond my experience. The point of connection is that I have become both; the point of difference whilst the analyst has dropped away, the Druid has not.

Until not so very long ago, I put both these experiences in the same category, as well as connecting them with the recurring childhood dream, recounted above, and a vision of a flying saucer. This was not because of any obvious similarity of content, but because they were all seemingly and similarly strange. So, I had collected and put them in a kind of *psychic* category, being immaterial and unexplained, and not connected to my daily reality and experience. Interestingly, I chose not to share these experiences with anyone, particularly in my family. This was not because of any question about my sanity, it was because it felt I somehow should not.

At the aforementioned time of professional and personal confusion, I was swept along by a wave of synchronistic happenings into the therapeutic chair of a Jungian analyst, although not a medical one… and a woman. I didn't want to train; I just wanted my mind sorting out. I now remember that in the many years in that said chair, I do not recall sharing any of these experiences. Strange, Jungians like that sort of thing. But I did eventually train: I was encouraged, cajoled, and finally acceded. My soul had awoken and was being nurtured, and psychoanalytic training seemed to offer a resolution to the impasses of medical and psychiatric specialisation. Some years later I qualified as a Jungian psychoanalyst.

I feel that the childhood visionary experience somehow guided me in some way, because I also now see it as different from the others, including the experience of the Druid. It still has a memory content, in that I can recall when I saw the figure of the psychoanalyst in my visionary imagination, I recognised it was something about my future, although I did not actually associate the vision with my training and qualification experience. It is only now, when alchemy rather than psychology has become my mainstream – rather as it did with Jung himself – that the visionary association has been made, and my formal position as a psychoanalyst has dropped away.

Maybe the vision was intuition and I was reaching into the future, extracting or seeing something to guide me. Maybe this is where the connection with falling in love comes into play. After all I was about twenty-eight years old, the time of my astrological Saturn return, and my life was going through a significant and sometimes dramatic reorganisation. I had left my marriage and wondering what the hell I was doing in the medical profession. I was drinking too much, and also driving too fast; literally, as well as metaphorically. Now I see this all a bit differently, I see that the time of the original vision was irrelevant in its linear capacity. With my newly awakened or discovered soul, I started to see time separate from space, and that this complex of experiences – past, present and future – were actually wedded altogether and somehow existed within the present.

Somewhere in all this is the timeless present, appreciated by the awakening of my soul. Falling in love is possibly good psychic therapy, although if one is married with a family it represents a deep moral challenge. Into this context I can see the psychoanalytic experience of my childhood. So, what about the Druid one? By contrast, this never had the quality of the present, nor did it seem to intersect directly with my personal and cognitive timeline, which the psychoanalytic one had. At least the latter taught me to see the purposefulness of memory and its attendant emotion; sometimes painful to face, but important to integrate into some sense of personal unity. Although there were some similarities, the Druid experience did not comfortably fit this category. It was more distinctly timeless and, if I give it a more transpersonal quality, it was from a more distant past, maybe even an ancestral one. Yet it was also intersecting with my present, although less with a memory quality and not one I readily identified with myself in the personal sense, even though that is included somehow… as I did subsequently become a Druid.

The experience of falling in love (though the relationship ended during my therapy), my therapeutic analysis (that is, myself being put through the ringer… or analysed), and my gravitation into mental health practice (though retaining an avenue in physical medicine), led me onto a different path. It felt that my soul had awoken and that I was now pursuing a kind of parallel path to the one that existed in the day-to-day world. I managed this reasonably comfortably, helped (maybe) by alcohol, whilst facing various health and personal challenges. Then the Druid started to awake.

But before I get to him, let me take stock with a couple of issues raised here: Why have I introduced this personal experience into this work? As this will be a central perspective in exploring Merlin, maybe some explanation is in order.

Most works on Merlin fall either into the factual or fictional categories. However, the former is often used as a surreptitious scaffolding for the latter, whilst the latter often influences the former. This can be in a mixture of ways, be it personal bias or mythic reconstruction (I will get to this a bit later…). A lot of this could be clarified if the writer showed his or her hand and with it any bias or prejudice, although it is seemingly understandable why they do not take this route, and for many reasons or justifications. The whole issue of lack of awareness or unconsciousness clouds this issue, so I am taking another approach.

Emotionally, writers are attracted to Merlin. I certainly am, so I want to outline why I am and hope that my biases will be readily available to see. Because these biases will inevitably cloud any reader's judgement of my approach and conclusions. This may work as an authorship technique, but nor for the kind of exposé I am seeking. Maybe that isn't exactly the point though: It is questionably more important for me to demonstrate my personal connection with the factual, mythic, archetypal figure that is Merlin, warts and all. In so doing, I hope to flesh out a different figure and one that we can all more readily relate to, even identify with and draw upon for the challenges that face us in the present.

In identifying myself in this archetypal complex that is Merlin, I also intend to draw upon the psychic energies associated with it and use them creatively and purposefully. This work is one such attempt, although other avenues will be apparent in my account. I contend that the rediscovery of Merlin is within our own psychic make-ups first and foremost, and any meaningful reconstruction flows from this. This more collective realisation, and with it the intent, purpose and direction of this realisation, I trust will become apparent. Because in the manner in which I am treating Merlin – vaguely but not necessarily accurately Jungian – I feel he is a significant archetype of our time and in urgent need of restoration.

The second issue is the complex one of memory. In the modern era memory has been given a more psychological and specifically cognitive understanding, but remains somewhat elusively outside of our grasp. If that were not the case, then the incomplete grasp of and paradoxes inherent within areas like post-traumatic stress disorder and repressed memory syndrome would not be so problematic. Also, I don't believe that the broader depth psychological findings of the last century, stemming from Freud and inclusive of Jung, fully answer these difficulties.

We commonly see memory associated with the mind, which the Latin origins of both words do so incline us toward. However, when memory is associated with the verb *remember*, then another line of inquiry opens up. *Member* can mean a *limb*, and so remember means to bring the pieces back together or, in modern metaphoric parlance, to make whole. *Remind* could be similarly considered. It is this more literal as well as spoken verbal and fluid function I want to pursue, because memory as a noun is somewhat static. Memory leads beyond a purely scientific and hence cognitive approach into a quality of our consciousness that is itself fundamentally beyond cognition, the brain, and even the body.

The quality of memory that links the two cases of my early childhood experience are not primarily cognitive, they are more emotional, which then relates to a feeling evaluation and discrimination. I have progressively inclined to see them in a context outside of the space-time continuum as we commonly conceive it, and to be autonomous, powerful, and directive. These are all potentially archetypal qualities. And it is emotion that has led me there, not cognition. Memory is powerful because of its emotional content; that is its power, it is seeking to be heard and integrated... made whole. This is the wisdom that stands beyond the apparent disorders such as post-traumatic stress disorder.

From an alchemical perspective, what I have done is shift the emphasis from material reality; I have not ignored the latter, I am simply pointing out its limitations. Material reality is practical and *earthy*, reality and sensate-based. It is bound by space and, to a lesser extent, time, providing us with the tools to survive and procreate. But we are more than this, and this 'moreness' will unravel further as this tale is told. Here, the shift has been to another of the primal elements, that of *water*. Hence the emphasis on verbs rather than nouns, which describe process rather than structure. And hence also accounting for the fluidity inherent within our mental processes, or psychic reality.

As an aside: I do not see the *psyche* as equivalent to the mind; the latter is generally more cognitive, earthy and material bound, whereas the psyche is greater than this. In the individual it approximates to the *soul* and collectively relates to *spirit*. Where I use it, I will incline to adjectives such as psychic and psychical, rather than the confusing Greek word Psyche; mind can be confusing in a different but not dissimilar way. Both terms – psyche and mind – we tend to equate with our cognitive and material selves, which we find difficult to define in the body, yet also experience more metaphysically or *beyond* the body, although connected with it. This connection is considered generally via the brain, to which we then give superior qualities over and above other bodily organs, maybe most specifically and relevantly the heart. There is no getting away from the obfuscation in all these terms, coming as they do from multiple language sources and tempered by our own cultural and personal preferences. I will try and negotiate this minefield by using some of this terminology, but defining the way in which I see and use it.

That was a bit of a detour, but with Merlin there is some difficult, complex, and confusing territory to cover. It is best if I play my hand, so to speak, not only in the way I am tackling the subject, but also where my approach is at variance to that of others. Personally, I believe any study of Merlin demands a difference in the way we have been looking at it and him, to date. The reader may not always agree with me and I don't pretend to always be right, but I do intend to provide and make a *difference* in the way Merlin is inquired about. And fundamental to this inquiry, I start with myself and my own experience. So, back to my Druid memory.

The psychic experience that I refer to as my psychoanalytic memory can be described as a personal or subjective one; that is, it associates with a linear timeline and has some cognitive features that we routinely associate with memory. What I am suggesting here is that by stretching cognition into emotional and intuitive realms – which can still be seen as some sort of continuum with mind-as-memory – there is a fuller sense of the experience. But this requires irrational functions, such as intuition to be included, as well as giving a primary importance to emotion.

The Druid experience is both this, and much more. I also see it as more transpersonal and metaphysical. However, I find both these terms problematic, as they tend to exclude the personal and physical respectively. A genuinely holistic appreciation is *both* personal *and* transpersonal, or personal:transpersonal according to my earlier terminology. To my understanding, psyche is also inclusive of the body, in a way that our modern understanding of mind and body tends to divide, separate, and split asunder. (I will be revisiting and explaining these points in more detail in the next section, *Bridging*.)

The Druid experience is beyond the personal and more objectively psychic. I contend it can only be understood by entertaining such concepts as hereditary memory or Jung's *collective unconscious*; the enduring appreciation of ancestry and hence lineage; maybe such problematic terms like fate, and even the Anglo-Saxon equivalent term of *wyrd*. I suspect legacy is tied up in here, too. Whilst our physical genetic heritage may have a place, I believe that, rather like the brain – which is but a physical organ in the body, after all – DNA is the machinery of these psychic forces and not their source, although somewhat paradoxically, also part of them.

All this gives a richer and deeper quality to my experience, although – rather like dreams – I contend that all personal memory may rest on a deeper, richer and more objective psychic stratum. Yet my experience also illustrates something else; that there is a dynamic interplay between the subjective and objective psychic experiences, because both are contained within it. I also used the psychoanalytic experience to illustrate in more detail how the personal and subjective interacts with the objective psyche and, even though it is relatively understandable at a personal level, it also has deeper more objective threads in it. After all it did – along with falling in love and some synchronistic occurrences – draw me to Jung and a psychoanalytic career, which then led me to alchemy and hence a way of approaching Merlin; a way that he himself would have used, I somewhat whimsically contend.

From a psychoanalytic career, I started to chart my life differently and parallel to formal medical practice. Jung's ideas spoke to me and I began to explore my own heritage in some detail, even whilst living in Australia where I *see* Merlin's future. This ultimately led me to becoming initiated in a Druid Order and to lead an existence more compatible with these deeper callings in my soul. Eventually and somewhat inevitably, this path was to become the mainstream of my life. And I felt that was somehow 'it' for me, but it proved not. I had fulfilled the Druid memory at a personal level, but something deeper was drawing me. I started to recognise that even leaving medical practice and mental health work were not final acts, but a step in finding another or deeper wellspring from which I could work with them. But beyond all this, I recognised that it was Merlin himself who was talking to me, taking me to task, and compelling me to get to the work that stands before you.

As stated, at first sight the Original Dream does not seem to be about Merlin. But it is, as my life is about Merlin, so I will outline how this dream started that journey. Because, at this time, the two prior memories were in my psychic data bank, but hardly at the forefront of my awareness. This dream, and the experience of stepping into Jung's work, would ultimately lead me to Merlin.

Whilst profoundly grateful to and historically influenced by Carl Jung, I am no longer a Jungian psychoanalyst. This influence permeates much of my approach to theory and practice, but there are many areas on which I beg to differ, such as with dream interpretation. I also feel that whilst he opened up the whole field of alchemy to modernity, particularly from an analytical perspective and understanding, there is much work still to be done as others like the analyst James Hillman have demonstrated, specifically in his work in *Psychological Alchemy*. My own approach is now idiosyncratic, but my feeling is that it was exactly this development that Jung had in mind with his concept of *Individuation*.

Earlier I described the recurring dream in my childhood. As indicated earlier, during this period I also had a flying saucer visionary experience. Interestingly, the night after the Original Dream of my analysis, I also had one of flying saucers. I have not had one since, although I have had psychic experiences of them separate from any visionary state, and I also have had an isolated abduction experience. I see these as clusters of psychic activity, when the opening between the worlds of daily reality and those perceived in altered states are more permeable and traversable. I now want to link these back to my experience of Merlin to this point in time of the dream.

I was born in the wake of Hiroshima. It was like a psychic pall that hung over my childhood, along with the indeterminate nature and outcome of the recent World War. This was not an immediate influence; I had more than enough on my hands with my own survival in the world and negotiating the more distinctly Freudian nature of family upbringing, a quagmire that occupied so much of my therapeutic analysis. But a personal world with conflict and a collective one out of war with an equally unresolved agenda, Hiroshima symbolised so much.

Maybe that is why the island was called thus? Without this, the early part of the dream is easily interpreted, but the juxtaposition of the peaceful Pacific and the cataclysmic event of Hiroshima made for an uneasy peace; a tension hung in the air. Although not of my personal and direct experience, it was as if Hiroshima was present within me as a memory of significance, as for many. Of no small interest to me is that many of the personal accounts of Merlin, particularly the vaguely historical Myrddin, were associated with the carnage and grief of the battlefield. Issues of blood, vengeance and retribution will continue to feature, particularly in the Grail accounts.

Not a lot of Merlin in all this, is there, with the exception of my association of him with the garden Druid? In the Original Dream there are only the vague glimpses around Hiroshima, and then some of my own personal association. This is more about me personally, although in a more Jungian and archetypal context where I am distinctly the observer. By the time the second part of the dream emerges – and it does feel to follow on from the first – I am more present and active. I am the doctor in practice, which at that time I was. It was the cornerstone of my life professionally, although personally my interests gravitated to the erotic discovery of being in love and the sexual exploration that was flowing from this. The dream was also now in a previously non-existent countryside; I was returning to my rural roots, something that the historical Merlin had recourse to do.

Julie was my receptionist in reality. Maybe more than my lover or my wife, she was compatible with all the dimensions of my life. Yet our relationship remained professional with a deeply personal undercurrent. And she was also from the West Country of England, one of Merlin's physical locations, if not the main one. I wonder now if this is a significance I had hitherto failed to notice, as I was more focussed on Julie's consummate professionalism and ability to make patients feel at ease. These subtle elements have dogged me and are maybe one reason the dream, now more as a memory, has persisted and pestered me down the years.

In many ways, Julie is like the alchemist's assistant who is also known as the *soror mystica*, a Latin term that literally translates to his mystical sister, or more metaphorically his *soul assistant*. The inference here is the balancing of masculine and feminine patterns and forces in the work of the alchemical process as reflected or actually mirrored between the two, such that they are effectively one and transcend any sexual or gender differences in the realisation of the goal, the making of alchemical gold. Lofty attributes, but are they valid? I suspect so, because this pattern is itself mirrored in the *original man and woman* in the dream. So, I will move to explore them a little more deeply.

Originality is a multifaceted word, which also has alchemical undertones in the base material that is to be worked with in the making of gold, and this was also the 'base' dream of my analysis. My suspicion is that the overlap with Christianity has obscured something else for me. I saw the prior *knowing* of the woman – beyond any sexual implications – to relate to Mary and the son to Jesus; God, the Father, being the unknown original male. But this has never quite fitted for me, mainly because the man both appears later in the dream, and also because there is something else implied within him: A distinct physical presence and as a sexual consort to the woman; neither are divine attributes in the Christian sense, although they may still be something paranormal or ancestral about him. This outlook is more alchemical.

But this also vaguely mirrors Merlin. He was born of a physical woman and an apparently metaphysical entity, an incubus if Geoffrey is to be believed. This story has been so Christianised that it is sometimes difficult to disentangle the accretions. These include Merlin's mother being a virgin, escaping death with her pregnancy, and becoming a nun. It also includes Merlin's father being demonised and identified as the Devil himself. The overlap and mirroring of the Christ myth is appreciable and are issues to which I will return. It also relates to my own birth and the circumstances surrounding it.

Does that make the known son in the dream Merlin, or do I peel back Merlin to reveal his father? Or is Merlin the father? Somewhat tangentially, Arthur's birth was psychically or magically engineered by Merlin, or is it a metaphor for the latter's own coming into the world? Is the Christian identity of son and father significant here? These questions are all valid, even if they lead to yet more. I have followed most in my inquiry of this dream and am left with a further quandary: How much am I the doctor, healer or alchemist, and is this all simply a reflection of my own intrapsychic work? Am I all these figures?

The man emerging from the mists – a very Celtic image – is tired, exhausted. I suspect now that this is me as I was a few years ago, some forty years later. I am going through a period of revivification or renewal, and the dress code of the man very much fits the image of the successful professional man. But I am not that anymore, and that fact in itself is rejuvenating, as implied by the alchemical elixir of life… maybe that is what is in the jar? And this father is subtly and definitively not the Christian father; he is human, all too human. He is me. Yet he is also Merlin. The

Merlin after the battles, and his madness in the forest, emerging from the mists of time in a modern guise. He is revealed here to me by medicine and alchemy, plus a distinct shamanic disposition.

These many years later, as I review the dream, the alchemical themes appear obvious and distinct. Of course, they were not so at the time, although my study of Jung would gradually reveal these. In a way this presupposes that such alchemical symbolism is a bedrock of symbolism more generally, as a kind of metalanguage, so that I would not emotionally lose contact with the dream and discover these features over time. Maybe it is our perception of time itself that is in question, as reconsidering it in ways beyond the linear and space-bound one may reveal more about these questions than any reductive analysis.

But whilst alchemy as a tradition emerges strongly in the second millennium, is it correct to associate it with Merlin and possibly his heritage of Druidry? I will contend that it is. There is much in Merlin's story that is both shamanic and alchemical, which this work will attempt to uncover and reveal. I do not separate these two traditions to the extent that modern study does and, in fact, this account will do more to bring them together, if broader and a more archetypal viewpoint is taken. As a seeming aside and from a more personal line of inquiry in my researches, I have found the Anglo-Saxon, rather than the Nordic runes, to be of help with their connection to Christianity generally and the Grail more specifically.

The central theme common to Christianity, alchemy and shamanism, and hence magic, is transformation. Other terms, like rejuvenation and resurrection are associated with it, each providing a nuanced perspective. But the common feature, literally or symbolically, is the death-rebirth motif. It is present in the dream and could be tracked into any of the above three traditions, which I will be undertaking in various ways. It is in the *Charm of Making* itself. The central symbol or outcome of this process is the divine child, the alchemical gold, the elixir of life, or the unification of masculine and feminine. In the mystical tradition this is the Holy Grail, itself primarily derived from Celtic tradition and one reason maybe that Merlin persisted in the Arthurian and Grail legends beyond his apparent used-by date.

Underlying the emerald jewel is a fountain, a complex symbol mainly in the realm of the feminine. Present in the dream, supported by alchemical interpretation and a distinct feature of the Grail legends, the feminine is represented somewhat enigmatically in the female figures in Merlin's story. Some of this, of course, may be accounted for by patriarchal repression, leading to the mixed and varied accounts of Merlin's relationship with female figures and their somewhat contradictory stance toward him. But this does not fully account for the ambiguities, even ones inherent in my dream. Whilst resorting to mythology may help here, Jung's approach with such concepts as *anima* may also be of assistance. A deeper appreciation of the feminine is essential to both my understanding of the dream, the rather enigmatic conclusions to Merlin's earthly existence, and an appreciation of the Grail itself.

That, then, appears to be my task. To rejuvenate Merlin, in and through myself. That is the task that the dream has laid out for me. The Christian associations are valid, because Christianity itself tried to absorb Merlin into its story with Arthur and the Grail legends, where he could conveniently have been left at Arthur's conception. It will be necessary to honour these associations and their own necessity. There are many threads left loose and unanswered in this inquiry to date, but it is time to put them aside for a while. However, they will track through the unfolding account, even as I put the personal side of it to one side and leave it here.

Bridging

Before launching back into Merlin more definitively via Geoffrey of Monmouth's works, it is relevant here to provide a broader intellectual context in which the material to date can be set, which may then serve as a kind of mind-map moving onwards. There are a variety of disciplines that will resonate with such a map, and its strength is reinforced by this extent, familiarity and depth within such a variety.

The background to this mapping process is highlighted in the first paragraph of the preceding section and various comments I have made elsewhere, to date. The conundrum I am wanting to clarify – inasmuch as that is possible – is presented in my use of a colon to bring opposing words, like *body:mind* into some sort of unity. It is also symbolically present in the subtitles to this whole work. The *Creation of Merlin* is not directed toward a material and physical creation, although in literary form his creation into our minds took firm root with Geoffrey, by following his traces in earlier oral tradition. Also, the *Secret of The Grail* is not a revelation of something hidden or stowed away into the light of day, but a metaphor for what it represents to us that is presently obscured, and by what may become clear in what follows.

This is all made more difficult to appreciate in modernity, where our factual and data-driven existence has rendered concepts and ideas into a reduced and material categorisation, where even myth has come to mean the opposite of its authentic meaning. We seem progressively unable to live with ambiguity; we have lost an appreciation of analogy, metaphor and their symbolic bedrock in our language that is bastardised with acronyms and abbreviated text messages. We need to wind back the clock more than a little, otherwise the questions posed by *Creation* and *Secret* will remain unexplored and hence unanswered in the terms of reference intended.

Language, it seems, has fallen victim to our rational and masculinised consciousness; at the physical level of the brain, it is usually and predominantly located in the so-called masculine left cerebral hemisphere. Mentally dominated by cognition in various ways, we tend to take a material ('seen') orientation at the expense of the immaterial ('unseen') and analyse it with various functions such as causality, quantification and reductionism. We look at things abstractly and most particularly dualistically: White is white and black is black, under which we list things like good and evil, masculine and feminine, love and hate, light and dark. There are no shades of grey. Yet this does exist when we start to appreciate the co-existence of the opposites, as with day and night, and their interpenetration. We may all have experienced something we are told is good, to find it as being not so, even bad or evil.

The Chinese symbol *Yin-Yang* demonstrates this with a small circle of black being present in a sea of white that flows into the black sea and its contained small circle of white. Opposites flow into each other, they interpenetrate. The seeds of one is in the other and we cannot appreciate the whole without embracing both white and black. With reference to language, we have moved from a position where opposing views provoke disagreement, even argument, through to one of discussion and debate to dialogue, which after all means 'through logic'.

Yet we remain in the realms of rational consciousness with this step ('through logic'). Does it hold for *body* and *mind* of body:mind, which we struggle to see in such a simplistic oppositional way? Can we even take body and mind onto an equal playing field, as disciplines like medicine try to, even latinising it as *psychosomatic* to obscure the problem? The issue is: We can't. The body is physical, material, biomechanical in its essence; the mind is more mental, immaterial and energetic. Of course, there are areas of overlap and connect, such as the immune and hormonal systems, and with nervous functioning, particularly emotion; but essentially we see that the separate body and mind are somehow of a different *order*, as in a class or system, and cannot be so simplistically connected. They are certainly not simple opposites.

Given the earlier discussion about my childhood experiences, it may be appropriate to explore the terminology that psychology provides in connection to forgetting:remembering. The remembering aspect has been covered; *forget* and *forgetting* are equally challenging. The origins of 'forget' are Germanic, as in *for* (as in 'neglect') and *get* (as in 'retrieve'); so 'neglect to retrieve'. Of interest is that the word *forgive* is also closely related.

There is the more obvious cognitive forgetting, as with where reading glasses have been left. This is commonly because other issues are intruding, supervening or otherwise occupying or detracting from daily consciousness; cognitive impairment (for example, as in dementia) is also obviously an additional factor, but one I am not inclining here. However, this begs the question as to what these 'other issues' are, as they are obviously demanding to be *heard* and maybe integrated into our daily consciousness. This may not be as easy as it sounds, because the issues may be incompatible with consciousness and emotionally connected to traumatic events, real or imagined. In this case forgotten issues may be remembered only when in the state that they are associated with, demanding psychological or shamanic techniques to bring them back into daily consciousness.

There is also a realm beyond where things are forgotten, never or needed to be retrieved and remembered. This vast storehouse of events and experiences may be forgotten, but not lost, and may merge into information that we already carry within us – a kind of psychic DNA maybe – from our family, cultural and racial backgrounds. It was this realm that Jung was keen to explore and promote; a *collective unconscious* that exists beyond the *personal unconscious* of personally forgotten memories, which take on dark connotations when traumatically neglected and repressed. Jung saw these personally forgotten memories that are the consequence of trauma and conditioning to comprise the *shadow*.

More pertinent to the ongoing inquiry are the realms of the sexes. In the world at the physical level is *man* and *woman*. So far no problem, the differences can be seen as the small circle in the Yin-Yang symbol, but the two are of the same order in terms like quality and magnitude. But what about the less material and more abstract principles of *masculine* and *feminine*; are they of the same order, or somehow different, like the body and mind? This may take a little more to unravel, but it is central to this inquiry, most particularly when the Grail emerges for consideration.

Whereas men and women contain features of the opposing genders to varying degrees – and so comprising the rich spectrum we are negotiating in gender politics, sexuality etc. – the masculine and feminine principles represent the pure qualities of each as a kind of psychic blueprint or psychological prototype or archetype. Each of these archetypes can take on more specific representations; for example, the masculine could be the wise man, warrior, eternal child, priest or magician. Is Merlin an example, image or representation of such an archetype, and are his various historical contenders for his name or title people who at the personal level carry many of the features we attribute to him? Is this a general principle?

What I contend is that is the case. It is also apparent that our modern consciousness is and has been, for most or all of the two thousand years, dominated by various aspects of the masculine principle; in contrast, the feminine has been denied and repressed, particularly if it challenges the dominant masculine principle of the time such as the patriarchy. The consequence of this is that our daily consciousness is more masculinised subjectively and hence objectively (I will return to objective:subjective), and the feminine is more psychologically unconscious.

But is this a position that has always held sway? Many disciplines would tell us it is not and in my appreciation of them, the Arthurian and Grail legends are replete in this, as well as indicating that the feminine is traditionally more grounded in these deeper psychic strata, as her biology and psychology would indicate to many. The proximity to birth and the body is more immediate and profound, and maybe death and sexuality follow suit? My own researches indicate that the concept of *Soul* is more feminised, not only in men (as espoused by Jung), but in women as well. Maybe this is represented by one such as Merlin, who seemingly walks between these worlds and who has an enigmatic relationship to the feminine, such that he does not present in a sexually masculinised manner, which Gandalf certainly does not.

With this appreciation, the inquiry is becoming more deeply psychic and subjective. I contend that any psychology that explores these realms takes such a stance. So, in the objective:subjective dyad, maybe subjectivity matches the feminine and gains a depth of appreciation beyond the masculinised consciousness of the objective and material. Maybe – now here's a thought – our reality-based objective worldview is actually *constructed* from the subjective?

If so, we need to look at language somewhat differently from the restricted basis we presently do. It is not strictly reality-based and objective, but also expressive in analogy, metaphor and symbol; an alternative reality that the poet appreciates, maybe with 'his' more feminine nature, women poets notwithstanding. History (masculine) has its mythic (feminine) nature embedded in it, one reason these traditions and legends have held so much psychic sway. They may be as important to listen to as the historical; maybe even more so.

Finally, a numerical theme we touched on earlier was the difference between three and four; maybe this could be written 3:4? I am now moving from the apparent (I stress here, *apparent*) unity of our conscious awareness, or *one*, through the *two* of the dualistic or binary position elucidated in some detail above, to numerically expand into and include *three* and *four*. I have nominated four as representing daily reality in some way, which agrees with Jung's impression that four, in a quadrated pattern like compass points around a circle, is how the greater metaphysical reality somehow *manifests* in the spatial world and our individual consciousness. So where does that leave the number three?

In my view, and in a way that draws Celtic parallels and the importance of the triads and other creative forms, the number three represents the physical, the metaphysical *and the ground between*. It is like process or fluidity – water even – as opposed to structure, form and the fixity of the world. If we now propose a *great binary*, being *self:spirit*, then this third intermediary point is the rather ethereal *soul*, which is *both* personal *and* transpersonal, or collective: The either-or division has dissolved.

As a brief aside: Many commentators deal with these seemingly irreconcilable opposites (irreconcilable, because their inherent natures differ so greatly rationally), by providing a continuum or spectrum, as in the Perennial Philosophy (of Aldous Huxley and others) or as a Spectrum of Consciousness (Ken Wilber). These are recognisable as body-mind-soul-spirit in New Age circles, and can be expanded to provide more in the way of connecting points and thus an expanded spectrum, by including emotion somehow (I will return to this area). The more concrete representations of mind and soul can be viewed as brain and heart, and then subtly as the functions of thinking and feeling. Personally, I find all this becomes cumbersome and the psychological self to include the body:mind, so I prefer the triadic simplicity implied and embedded in the binary of self:spirit. I will return to this conundrum in Part Two, where the issue of the Son of Man and/or God will present itself.

Soul, as intermediary, translates or mediates the daily reality from the metaphysical; it can relate to the marginal, the liminal state of being; it can be seen to be begun with a capital or small letter, depending on context. Life is created from the beyond or – even if metaphorically – death; the beyond also being the *home* of the archetypes, or in tradition the ancestors. Now it is worth reflecting back more deeply at the translation of the *Charm of Making* that begins this section, as well as the other originals that begin this work. It may also be appreciated where the dreams elucidated to date fit in. The concluding section to this work, *Merlin and The Grail in The Psyche*, will expand on and expand these issues further; at present, they are guidelines in which to approach the material that follows.

Before closing this section, there are a couple of points that are worthy of mention. The first is that emotion – meaning, literally, *motion out* – has a strong resonance to the in-between point of the *self:spirit* binary being the link between the self and spirit, hence a function of the soul. "Emotion is the vehicle of the soul" quoth Paracelsus, the great early 16thC physician and alchemist. Emotion is also related to the concept of energy manifesting into the physical, the body. As an aside, the *mind* remains merely a cognitive derivative of the brain and hence body, unless infused with emotion via whatever source; such as sexuality, drugs and creativity, to name but a few such channels (or portals).

The second is the role of ritual and creativity as being *states* in which this liminal or in-between space is accessed, and hence the beyond becoming manifest in that state. Traditionally ritual, through such agency as a sacred space (grove, medicine wheel, retreat etc.) and technique (meditation, dancing, chanting, drugs etc.) is used to create a liminal state in the individual and hence become a channel for any transpersonal and spiritual energies to emerge. Creativity is a specific channel that we all have the capacity to engage; indeed, Jung saw creativity to be an *instinct* specifically in man to accompany the four ones of fighting, fleeing, feeding and fucking that we share with animals.

This in-between state is the also the place of the magician; it is also Merlin's home, his *Esplumoir*. This will have increasing significance when I explore his later time in the world and what ultimately happened to him.

The Life of Merlin

History and Fable

In general, when we reconstruct the past we tend to do so from the information provided by history. As we know now more than ever, there are many distortions in this approach, but from a reality-based and objective perspective, we seem to have little else. Supported by disciplines like anthropology and archaeology, the view into the past retains this general historical and somewhat linear perspective.

In Geoffrey's creative period of 1130-1150, and shortly thereafter when the Grail emerges into the picture, England was still in a state of political and social flux. It was less than one hundred years since the French-Normans assumed power and when this French influence superseded the titular Anglo-Saxon period. It should not be forgotten that the Normans were originally Norsemen from Scandinavian stock (Vikings) who had settled in France, Normandy in particular. In this sense there is something of a continuity with the state of Britain prior to 1066, when the Kings were a mixture of Anglo-Saxon and Scandinavian-Vikings, although this particular change does seem to have been culturally abrupt. It was in this mixed culture that Geoffrey flourished, although his own background was Welsh and he wrote in Latin, which was usual at this time. He was also a Churchman, rising in rank as he aged and possibly ambitious in this sphere even, and somewhat interestingly, inclusive of his Celtic leanings. It was in this context that he conceived – gave *birth* to – Merlin.

Prior to the advent of a centralised Kingship in England stemming from the 9thC and the various Viking invasions over the next two hundred years, there were minor or lesser kingdoms, collectively known as a heptarchy, which gradually emerged after the Roman departure in the 5thC. It is in this post-Roman mix that Merlin flourished in a vaguely historical manner. This was in regions of England and Wales where the Celts were strategically pushed by the Romans. Scotland had and still has an enigmatic relationship with its southern neighbour, but had a strong indigenous population, being Scots (from Ireland) and the more obscure Picts in the North. Ireland was never colonised by the Romans, though the Church later rectified this apparent omission. With the more bureaucratic Romans and later the Catholic Church of Roman persuasion that superseded the indigenous Celtic version, pre-history starts to merge into documented history, which is now mainly in the Church's hands. Any accurate perspective into the distant past becomes progressively more obscure and prejudiced. Instead, we have to rely on traditional and folk input, including myth and fable; a heady mix indeed for those of a more rational persuasion.

If looked at in reverse, from the depths of pre-history into history and ultimately the present, it is probably wise to suspend rational belief and adopt a more mythic and imaginary perspective, or metaphysical sensibility to the present subject matter. However, sometimes it is difficult, though not impossible, to uncover this perspective from under the cloak of history.

The Irish situation can be used for some sort of comparison. There are fabled waves of invasions, probably vaguely representing real events, that preceded the presumed last, being the *Tuatha Dé Danann* or the 'Folk of the goddess Danu'. Maybe Scandinavian (Danish) in origin, the mythic origin of these people is the fabled *Hyperborea*. Existing in the 'far north of the world', Hyperborea is psychically linked to such fabulous islands as Atlantis and Lemuria. The Tuatha brought with them four *hallows*, or treasures – a cauldron, stone, spear and sword – that I will re-engage with in some detail later. Such invasions were mainly by sea and sometimes from less neighbourly and more distant lands than is commonly presumed. A feature to which we will return is the prominence of the sea, not only for the movement of people and hence culture, but also as a basis for the mythic imagination in contrast to the land.

The traditional foe of the Tuatha were the incumbent *Fomorians*, who seem to represent the more harmful aspects of nature. Put this fact – mother nature – together with the Tuatha being 'Folk of the goddess Danu', and there arises an interesting focus on the feminine as mother and goddess in this pre-historical period. I question what this has to say about the feminine and its pre-eminence, given that the Tuatha were considered to retreat into nature with the arrival of later more historical peoples, and then exist in the supposed *Faery World*. Maybe this is not just in our imagination – the soul is often considered feminine after all and certainly has feminine qualities – but somehow co-existent or interpenetrating our consensus reality. How far does this explain the common view of supernatural and paranormal phenomena?

Of significance to me here is that there is not a clear relationship with the Celts and the land, as we are given to believe in modernity. They, after all, arrived in Britain and Ireland from central Europe only 500 years or so before the Caesar's Romans invaded England later in the last century before the common era. With the notable exception of Ireland, a lot of this mythic material was later collated by the Church in its own idiosyncratic style (meaning: Can this be relied upon?). Alternatively, I favour a preceding Druidic history in this mix, or at least a sacerdotal religious class that *informed* the priesthood of the Celts, being considered as Druids in modernity.

In Britain, this mythic mix was most evidently significant in both Wales and Scotland, both of whom – although in differing ways – were affected by subsequent military and political events. After the Romans left, this mix re-emerged in Wales and Scotland and included myths and tales in oral narrative and later verse that included figures who resembled Merlin, such as the Welsh god-figure and magician Gwyddion. Yet Geoffrey had strong Welsh inclinations and heritage; it permeated his ancestry and hence his being, and so it had a formative effect on his writing and hence the personal resonances that exist therein.

Synopsis of the *Vita Merlini* of Geoffrey of Monmouth.

Vita Merlini, or *The Life of Merlin*, is a Latin poem written around the year 1150. It is now widely accepted to be the composition of Geoffrey of Monmouth. *Vita* tells the story of Merlin's madness, his life as a wild man of the woods, and his prophecies and later conversations with his sister, Gwenddydd, and the poet Taliesin, amongst others.

The plot derives from previous Celtic legends of early Middle Welsh origin about the bard *Myrddin Wyllt* (Myrddin the Wild), specifically a figure in Welsh legend. Another related legendary wild man was *Lailoken*, who was a contemporary of St. Kentigern (aka St. Mungo, flourished late 6[th]C) and lived in the Caledonian Forest in the Scottish Highlands, where he suffered a threefold death. Other similarly legendary appellations, such as *Silvester* or *Celidonis*, refer to his association with the Caledonian forest. Further to this, the related figures of *Ambrosius* and also *Emrys* have more southern Welsh associations, and they haunt me a little with their Romano-British, regal and Arthurian associations, as well as with their potential significance.

Vita also includes an important early account of King Arthur's final journey to Avalon, which is a little tangential and apparently anachronistic if connecting this Merlin of *Vita* to the mythic one in the earlier *Prophecies*. Though the *Vita's* popularity was not remotely comparable to that of Geoffrey's *History of the Kings of Britain*, it did have a noticeable influence on medieval Arthurian romance and has been drawn on by modern writers, myself included; somewhat paradoxically, *Vita* may prove to be more significant than *History* to contemporary viewing.

When reading this material, it is worth considering not only Geoffrey's personal position, as outlined, but what unknown psychological issues may also have been present; such as his ambitions, preferences and other unknown factors, like the nature of his relationships. A major one would be: What was his need in writing the *Vita* given the success of his earlier works that included a differing portrayal of Merlin, and why after a significant time period of about fifteen years? These questions would go alongside the known: being the dedications of the works; his religious status at the time; the surrounding political atmosphere, as well as the location and influence of Oxford as a centre of learning.

Some of these issues merge across the psychological *personal:collective* spectrum derived from Jung: Not only may Geoffrey have written *Vita* for personal reasons, but it may have been that the spiritual impulses within the material – desirous of not being lost – used him as a creative portal to achieve this. In other words, was he *used* for spiritual purposes beyond his personal ones? Did he lapse too much into the Faery World of his Celtic background and do their bidding? I am being far from trite here.

In this context, it may be worth reading and experiencing the synopsis as if it were a *dream*. This is one way spirit or the transpersonal psyche talks when the mind is relatively disengaged from the process. That means reading it in a liminal space, if possible, and see what additional creative and imaginal material presents.

So, to the *synopsis*:

> *Merlin is introduced by Geoffrey as a prophet and king of Dyfed in Southwest Wales, who takes part in an unnamed battle alongside Peredur king of Gwynedd, in Northwest Wales and Rhydderch king of Strathclyde, against Gwenddoleu king of Scotland, being the Southwest of the present-day country. Gwenddoleu is defeated, but three brothers of Peredur are among the slain, although the poem is ambiguous and they could also be Merlin's brothers. Merlin so grieves at their deaths that he goes mad and runs off into the Caledonian Forest, where he lives on grass and fruit.*
>
> *Other histories have variations on these apparent facts in Vita: Being the associations between these various men; some ambiguity around the slain brothers as stated, and some understandable location differences. The battle seems to be the Battle of Arfderydd, or Arthuret, in 573 CE in Cumbria, where Gwenddoleu was killed in defeat. Two interesting associations are the name Arthuret and King Arthur, and that Peredur may be the Welsh precursor to Perceval of Grail significance.*
>
> *The news of Merlin's whereabouts eventually reaches his sister Gwenddydd, alternatively anglicised to Ganieda, who is the wife of Rhydderch, and she*

sends an emissary into the woods to find her brother. The emissary finds Merlin lamenting the harshness of the winter, and responds by singing about the grief of Gwenddydd and his own wife, Gwendolen. The allure of this song soothes Merlin so effectively as to bring him back to lucidity and he is then encouraged to visit his sister at Rhydderch's court. Once he is there the strain of facing crowds brings on a relapse, and Merlin has to be chained by Rhydderch to prevent him returning to the woods.

When Merlin sees a leaf in Gwenddydd's hair he laughs, but refuses to explain his laughter, unless he is freed. When this is done he tells Rhydderch that the leaf got into Gwenddydd's hair when she lay outdoors with her unnamed lover. Gwenddydd then seeks to discredit Merlin by a trick. She produces a boy on three different occasions, dressed in different costume every time to disguise his identity, and asks her brother on each occasion how he will die. The first time Merlin says he will die in a fall from a rock, the second time that he will die in a tree, and the third time that he will die in a river.

Rhydderch is thus persuaded that Merlin can be fooled, and that his judgement is not to be trusted. Merlin is then asked if his wife can marry again, and he consents to this, but warns any future husband would need to beware of him. Geoffrey now explains that in later years the boy fell from a rock, was caught in the branches of a tree beneath it, and being entangled there upside down with his head in a river, he drowned.

Once again in the woods (although unexplained as to how he got there), Merlin reads in the stars that

80

Gwendolen is remarrying, so he attends her wedding mounted on a deer stag. Wrenching the antlers off his stag he throws them at the groom and kills him, but failing to make good his escape he is captured and taken back to Rhydderch's court again. There he sees first a beggar and then a young man buying leather to patch his shoes, and he laughs at each of them. Rhydderch again offers Merlin his freedom if he will explain why he laughed, and Merlin answers that the beggar was unknowingly standing over buried treasure and that the young man's fate was to drown before he could wear his repaired shoes. When Merlin's words are confirmed Rhydderch lets Merlin go.

Back in the woods, Merlin watches the stars in an observatory Gwenddydd has made for him, and he prophesies the future history of Britain as far as the Norman kings. Rhydderch dies and Gwenddydd grieves for him. Rhydderch's visitor Taliesin (a semi-legendary and contemporary bard) goes to the woods to see Merlin, and there he talks to him at length on a variety of learned subjects, including cosmogony, cosmology, the natural history of fishes and finally a survey of the world's islands, including the island of apples (Avalon) where Morgen tends King Arthur.

Merlin prophesies a little more, then reminisces about the history of Britain from Constans' reign to Arthur's. A new spring of water miraculously appears, and when Merlin drinks from it his madness lifts and he gives thanks to God for his cure. Taliesin discourses on notable springs around the world. On hearing that Merlin has been cured a number of princes and chieftains visit him in the woods and try to persuade him to resume the governance of his former kingdom, but Merlin pleads his advanced age and the delight he takes in nature as reasons for refusing.

A flock of cranes appears in the sky, prompting Merlin to teach them about the habits of the crane, and then those of many other kinds of bird. A lunatic appears, and Merlin recognizes him as one of the friends of his youth, Maeldin, who had been sent mad by eating poisoned apples that had been intended for Merlin himself. Maeldin is also cured by drinking from the new spring, and it is resolved that he, Taliesin, Merlin, and Gwenddydd will remain together in the woods, in retirement from the secular world. The poem ends with a prophecy from Gwenddydd detailing events in the reign of King Stephen (on the English throne at this time), and a renunciation by Merlin of his own prophetic gift.

Criticism

The figure of Merlin in the poem has been interpreted variously by different critics. He is hard to define and pin down, particularly as Geoffrey has changed his name, is relatively vague about his affiliations in the historical context, and is presumably conflating several narratives to suit whatever his agenda is.

Emma Jung (the wife of CG Jung) and Marie-Louise von Franz in *Grail Legends* saw him as a priestly figure, a kind of Druid or medicine man who "in complete independence and solitude, opens up a direct and personal approach to the *collective unconscious* for himself and tries to live the predictions of his guardian spirit, i.e. of his unconscious". This statement could be seen as shamanic; I will later contend that indeed it is. Nikolai Tolstoy found him to be delicately balanced between insanity and prophetic genius, so the psychiatric as well as the shamanic perspectives would be useful to explore. Carol Harding compared Merlin to a Christian saint, learned, withdrawn from the world, a worker of healing miracles, a hermit who becomes an example to others, resists worldly temptations and possesses supernatural knowledge and powers of prophecy; the end of Merlin's life, she wrote, is "a holy one in the sense any monk's is". I suspect this was Geoffrey's intention too, so as to remain in favour with his superiors, at least.

For Jan Ziolkowski his nature alternates between shaman and political prophet through the poem, ending up "as ascetic and holy as a biblical prophet". To which I add that there may be other possibilities in the ending, maybe mirroring his later Faery 'entrapment'. Stephen Knight's view was that Geoffrey makes Merlin a figure relevant to medieval churchmen, a voice "asserting the challenge that knowledge should advise and admonish power rather than serve it", is concise and accurate, certainly if Merlin is seen as a Druid. Mark Walker has written of the *Vita*'s Merlin as a figure at home in the romantic and humanist atmosphere of 12ᵗʰC thought, so sensitive that the death of his companions can bring on a mental breakdown, who eventually becomes "a kind of Celtic Socrates", so enamoured of scientific learning that he sets up an academic community where he can discourse with scholars of his own (and Geoffrey's) turn of mind, is very perceptive; I particularly like the association with Socrates.

(NB. This *synopsis* and criticism above is drawn from readily available online material, mainly Wikipedia, which I have tempered a little with my own comment, on occasion, to link this synopsis with my account, where relevant. I have read the original *Vita* in prose and found the above précis to be concise and accurate; any difference between this and other synopses are generally factual or interpretative, so being largely irrelevant for my purposes here.)

Elucidation

I will take the historical background no further; it will simply become more confusing. Suffice it to say that Geoffrey has eschewed the more pathetic version of the legendary Myrddin as a failed counsellor and negotiator, who loses his colleagues – maybe because of his actions – and ends up a lonely figure to be rescued by Saint Kentigern and Christianity, then to die a solitary death indirectly by a woman's hand. In this scenario, his madness may be a consequence of his culpability and guilt around the battle events, as much as any grief over the loss of either his lord or the three young brothers. But somehow, and maybe significantly and even prophetically itself, in Geoffrey's hands this narrative has become the background of something grander and more spiritually directed.

It is at this point that I realise how much attention I have paid Geoffrey and that for a while, with Vita still in my sights, I will continue to do so. I intend to pick up some of the themes in Vita and explore them, but leave others behind, as they are relatively irrelevant to my ongoing narrative. I have wanted to focus on Geoffrey because it was he who established Merlin in name and as a literary thrust into the future; effectively, Geoffrey is Merlin.

It would be interesting to explore Geoffrey and his intentions in the way the various commentators have indirectly in the above 'Criticisms', but that is not my further intention, except in a peripheral manner, on occasion. I have found it important to gain a perspective of him that, in a way, runs parallel to my own intention, as portrayed here. I have chosen Merlin as a significant background figure, even an archetypal one, to my own exploration and it is my contention that Geoffrey did as well, although for different reasons. I will have cause to revisit Geoffrey when his earlier Prophecies come into the account and some of the conclusions that arise there will help gain a deeper perspective of his contribution to Merlin's story.

Yet the Prophecies do get some attention in Vita. Merlin "prophesies the future history of Britain as far as the Norman kings" and "Merlin prophesies a little more, then reminisces about the history of Britain from Constans' reign to Arthur's". The first quote is interesting because it provides a link back to Geoffrey's earlier History without directly naming it; although Merlin himself is a direct link. It is as if in the Vita Geoffrey is trying to establish Merlin more definitively by giving him a background and history of his own, rather than the rather isolated and somewhat mythically rarefied appearance he makes in Prophecies within the History.

The second reference is somewhat different in tone. Merlin 'reminisces' rather than prophesies, which he did prior, although no reference is made to actually what. The use of the word reminisce I find interesting; it could have been recall, for example, or even remember, if my earlier comments are relevant here. The period of reminiscence is very short, because if Constans actually reigned it would have been early in the 5thC. He has links, maybe directly by blood, to the Romans, even the emperor Constance who is also referred to as the 'King of England' on occasion. Is Geoffrey trying to confirm the Romano-British heritage in the face of the Anglo-Saxons contributing to the political events of his own time? In some accounts Constans has two brothers, Ambrosius (recall Nennius' account of Ambrose) and Uther Pendragon, the purported father of Arthur, both of whom are named as Kings, with Vortigern intervening at some point.

These features, as well as the obviously glossed Christian

overtones, make Geoffrey's intentions clear, as well as establish Arthur's heritage more definitively. Yet they paint an unclear picture at the boundary of myth, fable and history. What does transpire from this is the more solid association of Merlin with Arthur, which becomes further elaborated and is distinctly highlighted in Malory, following the intervening Grail legends, where the two themes are somewhat unified into one tale.

Yet more important to this account are the themes in *Vita* that relate to my own story as well as its expression within a fateful archetypal pattern, as defined by Merlin, particularly via Geoffrey. One reason I am giving Geoffrey so much attention is that I feel he does something similar with his own personal story.

I find the initial part of the *Vita* account of interest, because it is of a different tone to the remainder; it is more contextual and historic, although somewhat blurred. It also outlines a history quite distinct from the earlier 5thC Romano-British one of Arthur et al, being more British – Welsh and Scottish – with clearly defined locations: Quite different from the "reminisces about the history of Britain from Constans' reign to Arthur's'" of later in the story, though maybe linking the two around Merlin? Once again, the difference between the more mythic English account and the wider more historical and British one comes to the fore, although Geoffrey may be making some attempt at reconciliation, specifically here by nominating Merlin's own regal origins ("Merlin is introduced by Geoffrey as a prophet and king of Dyfed in Southwest Wales"), and more generally with the *Vita* as a whole.

Be that as it may, what I am attracted to is the madness that follows the grief of the loss of the three brothers. I suspect this also relates to the odd figure of Maeldin who appears later in the tale, and to whom I shall return. At a psychological level Geoffrey is portraying a madness that is induced by battle, trauma and subsequent grief. This madness is of a different quality to that we associate with psychiatrically-inclined insanity, such as schizophrenia, although the triggers may be similarly traumatic in nature: Madness has more of an emotional nature that illnesses like schizophrenia are usually devoid of; such madness can be delirious and frenzied, as in some aspects of Merlin's behaviour, like dealing with his ex-wife's new husband.

This is my own experience. Dramatic changes in my life and its direction are associated with trauma, and are often self-induced, but also sometimes beyond my immediate circumstances or control, except when viewed synchronistically. Not only is this something experienced in the present, but it is also – and maybe deliberately – provoking unresolved past experiences, ones neglected or forgotten. There is a sense in my experience that somehow the trauma and its triggering are a necessary complex of outer and inner events that lead to a death-like state, but ultimately to a potential resolution, even a transformation. There are similarities in *Vita,* as Merlin is often the agent of this chain of events in his actions and utterances.

In passing, I find it interesting that whilst the loss of his wife may produce a frenzied and maybe retributive act of apparent violence or maybe vengeance, it does not produce the grief of madness. It is also significant that the feminine figure he relates more strongly to is his sister. Instead, it is the loss of his connection to the land that results in apparent relapses; Grail and Waste Land presentiments perhaps? After the death of my partner, I took our infant children away from the city to live on a rural property and ultimately develop a more communal retreat: I even named the property Ganieda, as the resonances felt strong at that time... and still do.

There is the impression in *Vita* of things being very urbanised and even somewhat incestuous, when Geoffrey describes Rhydderch's court and its social life. In contrast, we do not get a detailed description of the forest, only the effects on Merlin and his association with the fauna, as well as other features, such as astrology. It is as if, following the initial trauma of the brothers' deaths, he had to leave civilisation and retreat to the wilds of nature; not only to restore his health, but also to submit himself to a process of transformation. This is what I contend trauma leads us towards – change or transformation.

There is a cyclic process in this that Merlin submits himself to each occasion that necessitates it, even though civilisation tries to 'restrain' him in proto-psychiatric fashion. He finds the need to detach from the accretions of society and convention, to place himself in nature and its vicarious and sometimes brute forces. Somehow this is more *real* and there he can undertake the journey past the death-like experience that trauma initiates, into a passage – call it the *night sea journey* maybe – for resurrection, or transformation. That this archetypal pattern is demonstrated here, with links to others who have undertaken the same journey, is one reason that Merlin is resonant with the Christian story and maybe acceptable to others, such as Geoffrey.

This pattern and journey is one I am familiar with; it is also clearly present in the *original man* image in my Original Dream. This is not to be pretentious or grandiose; it is archetypal, it is available to all: This is the deep significance of the Christian story and its resonance with Geoffrey's account. Geoffrey was a cleric, after all, and this could portend Merlin's transition into a significant protagonist in the Grail legends.

This same pattern is also deeply shamanic and interlaced with prophecy, although I contend that not all of Merlin's utterances are prophetic. "Merlin sees a leaf in Gwenddydd's hair he laughs, but refuses to explain his laughter unless he is freed. When this is done he tells Rhydderch that the leaf got into Gwenddydd's hair when she lay outdoors with her lover." This is not clearly prophecy, although the laughter could indicate the potential frenzy or ecstasy of an altered state of consciousness; it is also possible that it could be because he recognises that Rhydderch has been fooled, or cuckolded. However, a little later in the account he laughs again, and this is more clearly prophetic, "There he sees first a beggar and then a young man buying leather to patch his shoes, and he laughs at each of them".

This laughter contrasts with the grief that initiated his madness and withdrawal to the forest, so can be taken as an indication of the ecstatic state of consciousness that can be associated with prophecy. As an aside, it also indicates the frenzied aspect of madness that I elucidated earlier, contrasting psychiatric insanity that lacks these features and is thus expanding on Tolstoy's position, as in the 'Criticisms' section immediately above; it is thus more clearly shamanic.

This is reinforced by his astrological sensibility, as "…in the woods, Merlin reads in the stars that Gwendolen is remarrying". Further, "Back in the woods, Merlin watches the stars in an observatory Gwenddydd has made for him, and prophesies the future history of Britain as far as the Norman kings." Astrology is closely associated with prophecy. This is more evident in the actual *Prophecies* of Geoffrey, and further reinforced by other prophets, most notably Nostradamus.

More could be said of the elements, particularly water that is involved in his healing on one occasion, as with music on the first. The water is from a spring, reminding me of the fountain of my Original Dream. The woods (or, more correctly, forest) are the background for these sensibilities that, with Gwenddydd/Ganieda's assistance, becomes his home. It is as if to contact these sensibilities and the marginal or liminal state in which they occur, one has to be in a conducive setting away from human traffic and distractions. When such prophetic and other unusual utterances breakthrough in conventional settings, as in Rhydderch's court, they are seen as strange, even mad. Merlin is therefore restrained, readily reminding me of the modern straitjacket as a means for dealing with the insane.

Ultimately, and with Gwenddydd's help, he retires to an observatory in the woods. The final paragraph of the Synopsis contains some condensed information. The account of cranes and other birds is distinctly shamanic and prophetic in quality; he also has a significant companion-like relationship with a wolf (not mentioned in the synopsis), maybe as a shamanic *power animal*. The educational domain, that overlaps that of any mentor, healer or teacher... or all three in one (I have used this triad to describe my professional activities) is also clearly present.

"(I)t is resolved that he (Maeldin), Taliesin, Merlin, and Gwenddydd will remain together in the woods, in retirement from the secular world" is an interesting quaternary, if my earlier comments on the number four are considered. The pattern would please Jung, particularly as the distribution is 3+1 (three men and a woman), as he finds this especially significant and expression of the central archetype of consciousness. That this should occur in the 'woods' reinforces this, in that this represents the *unconscious* and the other deeper aspects of the dyads I elucidated earlier and will come to in the concluding *Psyche* section of this account.

"The poem ends with a prophecy from Gwenddydd detailing events in the reign of King Stephen, and a renunciation by Merlin of his own prophetic gift." We are not told what prophesies these are, although Stephen was indeed King of England at the time this work was penned; it may have contemporary significance, yet I find it enigmatic. The issue here is that Merlin foregoes his own prophetic gift; but does one have a choice with such gifts? It may simply be that he declines to be in circumstances that initiate it, or that being *beyond* such gifts is actually a stage in spiritual development: Eastern spirituality would contend this as so; Socrates' sage maybe.

Yet there is also a transition in that the prophetic gift passes to Gwenddydd/Ganieda. I wonder if that is because this is where the gift originally emanated from; that is, spirit acting through the feminine, which may be a reference to Merlin's soul as well. It also reflects some of the conclusions of my Original Dream, in that it is 'through' the feminine that we perceive our path, fate or destiny, men and women both.

Finally, there is the odd appearance of Maeldin, who Geoffrey refers to directly as a "lunatic". Elsewhere he uses the word, "mad", so I wonder whether he sees them as synonymous? Mad is a word of Germanic origin with a wide range of application, even in modern English. Insane means 'not healthy', which is one reason I associate it more with psychiatric states like schizophrenia. Lunacy is also Latin in origin, which is the tongue Geoffrey wrote in, but also associates madness states with the moon and hence astrology… and alchemy, an art and science indirectly referred to at various points in the narrative. Approaching extreme psychiatric disturbance and distress with these three terms of madness, insanity and lunacy, would seem to offer some points of subtle differentiation that psychiatry lacks in blanketing them together. Add craziness and there is another quaternary.

But who or what is Maeldin? There is a Maelduin or Mael Duin in Irish mythology, also the product of a mixed Christian-Pagan union, being born of a nun – a rather unusual event, at least publicly – and a warrior who raped her. Whilst an interesting resonance and could be seen as a transcription change, I do wonder; it both mirrors Merlin's mythic conception and events that will emerge in Part Two. My thinking also goes elsewhere, such as the similarity of the name to both Myrddin and Merlin. Din as a suffix, as in Woden or Odin, may indicate a godlike quality or ancestry, something ascribed to Merlin, maybe via Myrddin.

Whilst I acknowledge my preferences here, I do question Maeldin's appearance, other than to make up the archetypal 3+1 so beloved of Jung. My suspicion is he resembles the alternative versions of fable, including *Myrddin Wyllt* and *Lailoken*, described earlier. These figures have a more ignominious ending than the Merlin portrayed here, if the fables and poems are anything to go by. So, maybe Maeldin is Merlin's *shadow*, as in the Jungian description of the term? This makes sense to me; the central ordering archetype that Jung calls the *self*, is initially approached through integration of the shadow or the more nefarious and unacceptable sides of the personality. This integration is essential to wholeness, achieved through individuation, and attained via healing. It also includes the feminine, as Gwenddydd, and another, Taliesin. The last is a semi-historical and legendary figure of the region, often associated with Merlin. He is known more as a Bard, and may indicate Merlin's creative function. Whilst this is a Jungian take, it does map Maeldin's appearance well in Geoffrey's account. There is also "Maeldin... had been sent mad by eating poisoned apples that had been intended for Merlin himself". Not only does this mirror the madness, it also associates the two figures... and even resonates with Avalon (the isle of apples).

Of interest to me was that I finished writing the above and put my pen down – a metaphor in the modern era, of course – deciding to go for a walk and, in so doing, realised I had not included the most essential prophecy, the *threefold death*. In fact, apart from making reference to the prophecies, I had not examined them in any detail at all. And I won't be doing here with the exception of the threefold death, because I trust the several scholarly commentators I have read who say that most are borrowed from elsewhere, even other cultures, as in the prophecy of the beggar. As stated, I have some doubt about the lover prophecy, although it does seem to fit the narrative more and portray an interesting dynamic in the relationship that Merlin has with his sister, Gwenddydd/Ganieda.

In contrast the threefold death has a distinctly Celtic flavour about it and, maybe indirectly, resonates with other aspects of *Vita*, as well as my dreams and personal narrative to date. The threefold death also points back to the comments I made earlier about not only death and dying, but also the role of trauma. I have further indicated that death is the first of an archetypal triad of a process that I have named as death, underworld (or night sea journey, dark night of the soul etc.) and resurrection; this is often abbreviated to death-rebirth, but I feel this neglects an important step in our understanding in the process or journey itself that potentially includes the creative function of madness. This also points toward the important concept of sacrifice that will be touched upon here, but discussed in more detail later, in Part Two of this account.

"(T)he boy fell from a rock, was caught in the branches of a tree beneath it, and being entangled there upside down with his head in a river he drowned." As with a lot of the poem, there is little in the way of elaboration or explanation. It does vaguely resonate for me with the entrapment Merlin sustains in the hands of Rhydderch, as well as his final 'entrapment' by the feminine in some versions of his ending. In my thinking, it is hardly a threefold death, as it seems that the drowning is what killed the boy. Yet there is much evidence that historical executions and sacrifices were more elaborate and ritualised than is necessary to effect a straightforward death. Although such forms of execution may have been used to prolong suffering as well as for both political and public reasons, as in the later hanging, drawing and quartering of the medieval period, it also seems to have been more specifically for sacrificial reasons.

Bodies have been found in bogs with a noose around the neck

and other significant physical trauma. Indications are that these were sacrifices, as the victims seemingly came from the upper echelons of society and had stomach contents that included some sort of soporific or even hallucinogenic component. Bogs are also liminal spaces, connected to the underworld, so reinforcing the idea of sacrifice. Most are from before the Common Era, overlapping the Celtic period, but existing well before it. It should be recalled that the Druids were considered to officiate at human sacrifices. All in all, they appear to have an important religious function.

Maybe the boy's death is a dim reflection of such a process, although it is not stated whether this was an accident, suicide, murder, execution, sacrifice… or a combination. Water is revered by the Celts as a liminal place; one only has to consider images like Excalibur and the Lady of the Lake, replete in the Arthurian legends. Rituals are considered by many, myself included, to be an essential component of attaining an altered state of consciousness in the liminal space so created, that can then be explored in the specific context of the ritual. The presence of the elements may also be significant, water – a feminine element par excellence – is here in the boy's and bog deaths. Of course, fire and earth are used routinely as cremation and burial. Burning people, either in execution or sacrifice, in a large wicker structure is a supposed fabled habit of Druids. Air? Maybe the boy's falling.

Sacrifice, of course, does not have to lead to actual death. Yet it is an essential psychic component of any authentic change and hence transformation. The fear of death, however, will also prevent the steps necessary to effect change. These are features of my dreams and personal experiences to date, and there will be more to come in Part Two. In some ways the threefold death is rather like my dreams, which could be seen as connecting points and transitional in themselves.

How much of *Vita* is shamanic? Much, I would contend. Following Glosecki, the major features of liminality and techniques of ecstasy, or altered states of consciousness, are there. Also, initiation – through the portal of madness – is clearly evident, as are the various tools-of-the-trade. The fact the Glosecki does not directly include prophecy has been discussed earlier, yet it is a rather obvious product of the above earlier two features. An additional factor for me that supports this contention is the introduction of Taliesin to the company. Prophecy is included in definitions of shamanism by others, most notably for me in Socrates. Again, I see Taliesin to support the second aspect of Socrates' definition, the artistic; the remaining two of eroticism and healing I will come to directly.

In fact, the prophetic function is what looms large in *Vita*, even if only to indirectly support the earlier *Prophecies*, enticingly the product of Geoffrey's creative and poetic art. All other commentators I have read highlight prophecy as if it emerges from these other functions; I have found this to be the case in my own life. Its significance in religion in the Bible cannot be denied, if this is any indicator.

What is notable to me – almost by its absence – is magic. In my earlier analysis, only Matthews has included it in his definition of what constitutes a shaman. As others have noted, Merlin only appears to conduct two magical acts; that is, orchestrating the conception of Arthur, and the building of Stonehenge. Neither are present in *Vita*, so what to make of these and, indirectly, the role of magic in Merlin's life and more generally in shamanism?

The Arthur story is interesting, as it becomes relatively enduring and features prominently in Malory and the movie *Excalibur*. It is also notable in the actual *Charm of Making* as 'thy omen of making', which is uttered to good effect by Merlin in the movie. But is this an act of magic, or itself a transformation, and are the two therefore somewhat synonymous? Merlin actually separately uses the word 'transform' with strong intent in the conception scene *Excalibur*. I contend that they are synonymous, and that the process of transformation undertaken in the death-rebirth cycle is in and of itself magical.

In *Excalibur*, Uther rides the Dragon's breath and transforms into the 'shape' or appearance of the Duke of Cornwall, Ygraine's husband, to sexually attain Ygraine and effect Arthur's conception. Shape-shifting is an art supposedly employed by Druids; I know, I do. It is a subtle art, such as disguising oneself in public or social situations. This could be as *another*, as in the case of Uther, or even as 'a cloak of invisibility'. So is Merlin employing magic or simply using his art in instructing Uther, or have hallucinogens been employed? Maybe both. In this context magic's definition becomes somewhat slippery and is one reason I see it to define outcome with the process undertaken to achieve this, as much as it is possible to do this.

Maybe this is more apparent in the building of Stonehenge. The fable is anachronistic: Stonehenge was built millennia before Merlin's time; at least the Merlin of this present incarnation. This may be a distant memory of the use of arcane techniques in the building or that Merlin, or 'The' Merlin, has a longer 'history' than we have supposed. But the descriptions of the building itself appear technical and hence not magical, as we might suppose it. I am reminded of Freemasonry here, however, as well as alchemy. It also harkens back to an era of ritual and religion that we have lost any historical connection with, but still appeals to us imaginatively and spiritually.

Rounding off Matthew's definition of Merlin are his attributes as a lover. This is indirect in *Vita* and for obvious religious and censorship reasons; but Merlin is married, although Gwendolen is a somewhat peripheral figure superseded by his sister. His act toward her new husband seems violent, but does have a ritual ring about it. The Stag is a significant animal in myth, most notably the Arthurian legends. In this context the act seems more of a ritual or even the portrayal of an imaginative altered state of consciousness. Why would Merlin otherwise be 'stamping his authority' when he has previously acknowledged that his wife may take another husband with his relative desertion of her, unless it could be considered sacrificial. Sex and power are maybe foreshadowed here.

Rather, Merlin's consort appears to be his sister, Gwenddydd. Of course, this could be seen as incestuous and in an almost Freudian context, but I contend it is not so. Rather like Julie in my dream, it represents the feminine in a more spiritual context, which I have previously likened to the alchemical *soror mystica*. In spite of her dalliance with a lover – which may be merely an artistic contrivance for the prophecy that follows – there is little direct sexual reference. Interestingly, it is a leaf in Gwenddydd's hair that gives her away; this itself may indicate her connection to nature and hence the forest where she ultimately resides after her husband's death, so maybe there is a prophetic element here as well.

My feeling is that the relationship with Gwenddydd is essentially a spiritual one of an alchemical nature. I don't see it as overtly sexual, although it is also possible that 'sister' may be a euphemism and she be Merlin's lover, and the leaf in the hair he might have directly contributed to; then, of course, there is actually no prophecy. I am being a little whimsical here, but these issues portend what is to come; being the role of the feminine not only in Merlin's life but also the Grail legends, as with the rather enigmatic alternative rendering of Merlin's last years.

In this alternative entrapment scenario of his ending in *Excalibur*, Merlin does not directly renounce his prophetic gifts, Morgana as his assistant extracts these from him by using the *Charm of Making*. He is then imprisoned by her wiles in using the Charm against him. (Morgana, interestingly, is Arthur's half-sister here). I find the ending of *Vita* more authentic and spiritually accurate, as the various alternative entrapment scenarios are distinctly Christianised. There is a difference in being tricked or deceived, to a voluntary return of gifts to the feminine, from where they originally ensued, after all. There is also the consideration that this is a voluntary sacrifice to the Land, in anticipation of renewal or rebirth. More to come.

Finally, there is the theme of healing, which is intimately connected to shamanism by all the commentators I have drawn upon, with greater or lesser emphasis. To me, it is greater, as espoused by the emphasis I have given to Merlin's madness and reinforced by my own trade. It is very clearly present in the second part of the Original Dream, where the father/man begins to look more like Merlin, or at least *a* Merlin.

Following his grief-initiated madness in *Vita*, Merlin is initially healed by an emissary sent by his sister, who does this through voice and "allure of this song soothes Merlin so effectively as to bring him back to lucidity". Briefly wondering who this emissary might be, apart from an agent of Gwenddydd, is that it is creativity and music that restores Merlin. I find 'lucidity' interesting; it is clarity, rather than sanity after all. Is Merlin healed, or is he simply encouraged to step out of his madness to satisfy his sister, because "Once he is there the strain of facing crowds brings on a relapse, and Merlin has to be chained by Rhydderch to prevent him returning to the woods." Interestingly, it is then that the leaf in the hair incident occurs.

Almost in passing, it is necessary not to exclude the various animals, birds and fishes that dot the account. These have shamanic resonances in and of themselves. I find their significance a little obscure apart from this, except they are traditionally both agents of healing and employed by traditional shamans in their ritual and healing practice.

"A new spring of water miraculously appears, and when

Merlin drinks from it his madness lifts and he gives thanks to God for his cure" marks the second, and seemingly permanent healing. Although on this occasion Merlin also remains in the woods; is transformed to the prophetless sage; becomes the object of extended attention; and passes into history without apparent death. Rather, it may be the context as much as the method that separates temporary recovery from true healing; certainly, the transformative elements are more distinct in this second episode. Yet water itself may be important in a primary manner. It is elemental and associated with the feminine as outlined in the Arthurian associations, as well as recalling amniotic fluid, if a more psychoanalytic perspective is taken. But in this context it is not simply regressive; if it is at all, it is in the service of rebirth or transformation.

And there I would like to leave this elucidation. There is, in my opinion, a lot more that could be extracted from and revealed by further analysis of the *Vita*. Whilst I find Jung's psychology very useful and appropriate to the above task, I am more driven by its resonance with my own life journey and as portrayed in the second half of the Original Dream. I am aware there are some areas that have not been fully examined, as yet, such as the forces of sex and power. Gwenddydd/Ganieda and Gwendolen raise questions about these forces in *Vita*, as Morgana certainly does in *Excalibur*.

However, the whole domain of the feminine to which I will come in more detail than immediately above, will have cause to revisit these figures and their involvement in such powers. I recall that Julie, a *soror mystica* figure, was a kind of Gwenddydd, whilst my lover at the time – not present in the dream – is relatively absent; Gwendolen has only token appearance in *Vita*. Sexuality is inferred in the dream, as with the *vice*, which also allies with power. Maybe it is not so much a question of *sex:power*, but that sex is power.

Deductions

Preliminary and tentative though they may be, it is at this point I would like to make some deductions that have arisen from *Vita*, as connected or extended to my own story. In this process there are similarities and differences that I will continue to weave together in this work, particularly when Part Two is considered. What I am presently deducing is that my story is but one of many that seems to resonate with Merlin as some sort of archetypal figure.

I have chosen to call myself a Druid, but is Merlin also one? Certainly, history provides such a possibility that has been elaborated on extensively in modernity, but this is largely medieval and legendary, extending from the pen of Geoffrey of Monmouth. To begin this inquiry, I would like to draw on a modern revivalist Druid Order with which I have had appreciable contact in the past. This Order, as well as some others, gives a tripartite structure of Druidry (using their term and adopted by many, the alternative being Druidism) and being: Bards, Ovates and Druids. In brief, these are the creative, healing and philosophical branches.

Without going into detail about the correctness or otherwise of this more modern perspective of the Druid, what I want to draw attention to is that these three functions reflect, and are sometimes the same as the various characteristics of shamanism that I have drawn on from such varied sources as Glosecki, Socrates and Matthews in particular, when a broader and non-secular view of shamanism is taken; that secularity is shamanism being an exclusively Siberian phenomenon. What this leads to is that Druids are essentially shamans, and are maybe the Celtic equivalent of the more academically strict definition of the Siberian shaman. Given that Merlin has many of these characteristics, including those provided by the great scholar of shamanism, Mircea Eliade, I will lay the matter to rest at this point.

The issue of names, particularly as applied to the archetypal Druidic shaman, Merlin, seems initially confusing. I certainly found it so, realising that any historical perspective becomes increasingly unreliable in general when going backwards through the Anglo-Saxon era (circa 400 – 1066 CE, approximately); instead, drawing on myth, poetry and fables that existed in oral form only and were then committed to writing with significant degrees of Christianisation. This is particularly so in the period being explored, around the 5th and 6th centuries. Similar difficulties exist because of the different languages that were involved in this evolving situation, being Celtic becoming Anglo-Saxon (or the equivalent term of Old English in the literary sphere) with the significant input of the broader Germanic language group, as well as Christian commentators writing in Latin. In spite of these difficulties and with a fair input of inspiration, I think that some broad sense can be made of the pre-historical figure or figures that comprise the background to his literary birth as Merlin with Geoffrey of Monmouth.

Myrddin is the name that is most seen as source. He covers the two locational areas of South Wales, extending to the West Country of England, and the borderlands of North Wales, Scotland and England. Interestingly, Arthur is also associated with both, although more the West Country than the South Wales of Myrddin. In his southern location, Myrddin is seen as some sort of chieftain or king and here given Roman affiliations with Myrddin Ambrosius and Emrys. This nexus is the one that the various medieval legends have promoted with the positioning of deductionsthese protagonists as Romanised British against the invading or colonising Anglo-Saxons, where Myrddin provides a Celtic and Pagan influence that, most interestingly, sustains into the medieval legends.

Here we find the Merlin of *Prophecies*, usually embedded in Geoffrey's *History*, with its political significance for the time he lived in. Following Nennius, Geoffrey placed the prophetic youth there, but named him Merlin rather than Ambrose. *Vita* followed well over a decade later and now places Merlin, more resembling the Myrddin of apparent history, in the second location on the borderlands of Northern England and Scotland, a considerable distance away. Did Geoffrey do this as an act of contrition, to balance or rectify his earlier account? Was Myrddin still such a significant figure in Tradition that he felt the need to do this? Were there more religious, heritage and cultural motives on Geoffrey's part – he was Welsh after all – in doing this? These questions have already been raised and there are many more, but although *Vita* is a more plausible historical work, it is the Merlin of *Prophecies* that has seized the day in modernity. Was this Geoffrey's intention, or was he trying to somehow countermand this initial success with *Vita*? As already indicated, I suspect the latter and for reasons to which I will come.

The Myrddin of the North is more plausible and does not directly relate to Arthur, which the historical time factors would also argue against anyway. Here, there are many intersecting figures by name, even to the Irish Suibhne (or Sweeny) whose story strangely resembles that of Myrddin. However, there are some of these figures who stand out more than others. Myrddin *Wyllt*, or Wild, relates to *Silvester* of the woods, so are more descriptive of the same person. More interestingly is *Lailoken*, the rather wretched and shadowy counterpart to Myrddin, who mirrors much of Geoffrey's account. This is around the infidelity of the Queen, although the King is now Meldred, and the symbolic *triple death* that involves Lailoken himself in a quasi-executory death… or sacrifice (see later). As a slight diversion, I mention Meldred because of the similarity of his name to Maeldin in *Vita*, as well as Mordred, who was Arthur's son in the legends killed by his father after fatally wounding him prior to his journey to Avalon.

In many respects Lailoken is a strong representation of Merlin, as rendered, glossed and sanitised by Geoffrey. But to my thinking he points in a direction that is incompatible with the Merlin of the South with his Roman background, and his support of the British against the Anglo-Saxons. This northern Merlin actually connects with the invaders, as can be determined by looking at the mythic and symbolic elements that even Geoffrey recounts. Not only this, but he then becomes associated with the British shamanic god-king, Woden, and he to Odin of the Norse. I also note that many British royal houses sought to have Woden in their genealogy.

Have I gone too far here? I believe not, so I will provide evidence from the sources already mentioned, but with a symbolic and mythic sensibility rather than a factual and historical one. In essence, I feel that Geoffrey has made a substantial attempt to bring into some sort of whole the various historical and mythic strands that surround Merlin as an archetypally shamanic magus, and that this was probably his intention. In this, I believe he wanted to establish the Welsh and British – Celtic – background to Merlin and Arthur, based on Tradition, with which to inform the events of his time. In so doing, he provided a forward thrust that was quite momentous, subsequently encouraging continental writers in the ensuing Grail legends.

I accept Geoffrey's position of bringing together the various Celtic figures of Myrddin et al into a unified whole of sorts. This more British complex is situated in Wales and the West Country, with Roman extensions as Ambrosius and Welsh as Emrys, providing the background for what follows in the literary and political arenas. Myrddin of the North may be the same figure, or a different one if the name were some sort of title, possibly Druidic. Myrddin as Lailoken, Wyllt and Silvester are more descriptive and this, with the titular possibility, make it unlikely that there is any unity of one person in fact, but only in fiction. Such fiction is mythic and archetypal in the shamanic and hence Druidic sense, and encompasses the described characteristics of Glosecki and others. But it also features ritual, initiation and sacrifice as major and ongoing themes with the cycle of death-rebirth. In other words, the unity is in the archetypal shamanic complex that radiates out to various individuals who carry distinctive features of this archetype.

I will now proceed to highlight how this links to my own narrative, which I believe would be the case for many people, both historic – maybe as the background to Geoffrey's Merlin – and present. It appears that the excessive Christian influence ceased half a millennium ago with Malory, but has reappeared through the back door in modern times in epics like Tolkien's *Lord of the Rings* and CS Lewis' *Narnia*. As stated earlier, I acknowledge Tolkien's Catholic influence in his otherwise Pagan saga; in many ways he mirrors Geoffrey, the Welsh cleric. Like Merlin for Geoffrey, I also believe that Gandalf is Tolkien's alter ego. I have my own, read on…

I was christened and later confirmed in the Anglican Church of England. Over a generation ago, when I started public presentations and other delivery about the modern medical system that might create professional difficulty, I decided to create a pseudonym. I had been interested in my heritage and spiritual background for some time, as is evident in this work, so I decided to consult the runes in a ritual of divination. As a result, I chose the name Kennan Elkman and used it in publicly. The rune *Cen* is with a hard 'c' that I anglicised to *Ken* and then *Kennan,* as I had found this to be a possible historical Anglo-Saxon equivalent to the Scottish Kenneth and Irish Keenan. This particular rune has distinct shamanic associations, it also relates to blood, sacrifice and the feminine. Some years later, when I moved location and changed my medical practice, I found that I was now more known as Kennan than my christened name, so I decided to legally change my name to Kennan Taylor. Latterly, I have also adopted a spiritual name, Osman, that resulted from a transition through a similar divinatory runic process.

Apart from psychiatric designations such as split or multiple personality disorder and other possible diagnoses, each name-change of mine has occurred at significant transitional times – both personal and spiritual – where ritual has been employed, sacrifice (of the old) undertaken, and any transition effected through initiation. Essentially these were times of death, change and rebirth; trauma being a significant undercurrent and often instigator. The earlier dreams contain these features as they have significantly informed and my life direction, supported by other information from such realms of consciousness.

If I compare this to Merlin and his various names, then maybe my story makes more sense; they do to me anyway. Although my names are around myself as a single entity, Merlin's are unlikely to be, if history is any guide. Then again, maybe mine are not, and I am spiritually drawing on ancestral figures who have walked this earth. I now see my various names as somehow and indirectly incorporated in Osman, informed as they are by divination (or magic) using runes, the archetypal language of yore.

I now intend to apparently digress and explore the runes in a little more detail, inasmuch they pertain to my story, but also the wider significance of Merlin. I also believe that the runes, more as a divinatory and magical tool than a script, are both indigenous to the peoples in history I am referring to and also flesh out the archetypal characteristics of shamanism. I do not see them as some sort of proto-language, but as a spiritually inspired and directed symbolic system of communication and magical usage.

The runes contain a framework that contains many of the themes I have employed around Merlin, as well as providing points of mythic relevance and archetypal connection. They are associated with the time period we are exploring: Being the Celtic through to the Anglo-Saxon period; the era of Merlin and Arthur of pre- and early history; the Pagan heritage prior to and during early Christianisation; a spirituality that is immediate through ritual, ceremony and magic, and more.

The choice of the name Osman is my own and relates to the runes, as described above. This was a conscious choice, so I cannot claim archetypal direction, although there may be some divine inspiration. As a name, it brings the 4th rune Os – ᚩ – rune to the fore, meaning a mouth as in speech and with Woden or the Bardic tradition in Druidry. In the Germanic rune row, the equivalent 4th rune is As – ᚨ – that relates to the Old Norse (ON) god Odin. There is a distinct tendency in the Anglo-Saxon runes to demythologise their Germanic cousins and use non-human symbols, associations and meanings.

As an aside: It should be remembered that the auditory sense was more significant in this era, certainly than in the modern era when the visual is now more dominant. The runes do have a pictorial representation that is of importance, but the *meaning* of the rune, including the glyph, was probably of more importance than we recognise. The bardic tradition had a significant social function, extending to the political and religious. There are also magical and other esoteric considerations, as exemplified in the word rune itself, meaning *secret* or *whisper*. Music and poetry are extensions of this function, so the association with the 'mouth' with the god of poetry and of pre-eminence.

Osman comprises two runes, *Os* and *Man*. *Man* corresponding to its Germanic equivalent - ᛗ. It is as the modern phonetic name implies, although the glyph is an image of two figures united, by a kiss maybe? There is symbolic significance to this; being the alchemical gender unity of the masculine and feminine, so Man is a generic term for both a man and a woman.

Of further interest is that I consider the name Lailoken to mirror that of Loki, the trickster-god of Norse mythology; the trickster being a further acknowledged shamanic characteristic. Loki is Odin's nemesis, and in Jungian terms he could be seen more as his shadow or dark side, although Odin has more than enough shamanic characteristics of his own with several other alter egos. Is Lailoken the same for Myrddin? Is the threefold death of Lailoken on the ash tree a resemblance of Odin? Is Myrddin, in fact, Odin or Woden?

I would contend that the association is at least strong. Their names have a similar – if not the same – suffix and *-din* may refer to a god-man. We are well into mythology here, so I will go with the flow. *Wod*, as in Woden, usually refers to inspiration, shamanic and divine, as well as elemental air. But what of Myrddin of the same suffix: Does the *Myr* refer to the sea, and water, so significant in the story of Merlin with its feminine presence and significance, as well as water as element? Are Woden and Myrddin some sort of masculine-feminine dyad, some kind of alchemical unity?

I will leave this inquiry there at this point. It may be quite speculative, but I trust it more than adequately demonstrates that there are other lines of inquiry that can flesh out the character of Merlin. It is simply that it is more productive, in my view, to take a more archetypal perspective to see how that various personages or alter egos of one person satellite around Geoffrey's 12thC construct of Merlin. But more than that is how my own story could be seen to connect with this.

However, the inquiry does not stop here and the prior reference to alchemy is not idle. A significant difference between the Germanic and Anglo-Saxon runes is number. The Germanic runes commonly number 24 and seem sufficient for phonetic purposes, but the runes are much more than this. In the latter part of the first millennium the more Scandinavian branch of Germania developed a contracted row numbering of 16, considered for more exclusive magical purposes and less available to common usage. By contrast, the Anglo-Saxon rune row progressively expanded, ultimately reaching 33; although there are variations on the specific number.

This increase cannot simply be explained by phonetics or script. Instead, I contend that it represents a divergence of Anglo-Saxon spirituality from its Germanic cousins prior to Christianisation and continuing through it. In particular, the latter runes from 28 on are distinctly spiritual in inclination, containing themes that, to my understanding, make use of alchemical themes and even Grail-like images. This operates as a kind of undercurrent to Christianity throughout the whole Anglo-Saxon period, alternatively it could be seen as a developing esoteric and mystical branch of Christianity. This may have had distinct Celtic Pagan influences, even a melding of sorts, prior to the strong arm of the Roman Church progressively asserting its more exoteric agenda. Maybe this is the undercurrent that flowed into the pen of Geoffrey and others in Merlin and the Grail legends; maybe Merlin had a hand in this development, reflecting his ongoing presence in the Grail Tradition.

I would like to stress that there is no extant evidence of Merlin being associated directly with the runes, although they are a short step away from the charms uttered by Merlin in *Excalibur*; the word rune does, after all, mean secret, and is definitively associated with Odin/Woden. In some respects, these runic changes and developments mark the birth of an England from its prior Celtic, Anglo-Saxon and ultimately Viking input prior to 1066. A little whimsically maybe, but Merlin's magical involvement with Arthur portends the birth of a nation; maybe he succeeded in this magical charm, after all?

However, the runes remain somewhat obscure during this period, enigmatically cropping up in inscriptions and archaeological finds. They are not directly present in Excalibur, which I find unfortunate, but hardly surprising with the more Celtic and specifically Irish emphasis. The interest here is mine, extending from a book I have written on this subject, and the association with the subject matter to hand remains that... as are the deductions I make from these possible connections. Irrespective, I find them intriguing and tantalising. These questions and the runes will be returned to in Part Two.

Winding Up

Orientation

By now it must be readily apparent that I use what appears a mixed writing process, which is generally rational and linear at one level, but well informed by associative thinking and bringing into the picture seemingly irrelevant material that I have given credence to, and attempted to justify in the process. Such an approach is holistic in the genuine sense of the term; not only associating known material, but also adding in speculative insights and finding with their undercurrents, known and unknown.

This is a marginal approach, in itself liminal much in the way ritual can be. This very work is a ritual; when I write I move into a slightly altered state of consciousness and draw on the ideas, imaginings and images that crop up to lead and direct me. I see such a positioning to have relevance; indeed, it must if I am able to write and what is written makes sense, even if the content may be under question for other reasons. Such an approach is cognitive at one level, with all the parameters that support this, such as causality, reductionism, quantification, dualism and others. Yet there are others we can relatively ignore, and my way of looking at holism includes the above parameters, attempts to unify them, but adds more abstract thinking, as well as associative connections that seem loose and emotionally driven – which they are.

Because I do not discount emotion, I include it in a

fundamental manner. From here I explore feelings, intuitions, evaluations and the like. Yet I retain the middle ground, the in-between state that liminality describes. The outcome I see as being an expanded and more creative way of dealing with the material, as well as extending beyond the historical, literary, archaeological and other disciplines we readily and sometimes over-exclusively draw on. I further believe this kind of *middle ground* is a soulful position, although not the only one that can be adopted.

The soul also has a presence in the body, as experienced energetically, particularly sexually. There is also the one that Socrates describes in relation to characteristics described earlier attained through an ecstatic state, which he describes as *daimonic* and hence closely related to madness. The daimon, or genius, is something I will be revisiting when Merlin's enigmatic birth is recounted. The importance of this is that it is this latter soul-state in which the shaman travels in psychic reality, such as in soul retrieval healing work for others, who have lost theirs.

This middle ground soulful position permeates *Vita* and there is more to come, particularly in Part Two. By taking such a position, I find myself *listening*, in the sense that there are undercurrents that seem to talk to me that I can sometimes identify as personal, with the preferences and subjective material that is inevitably included, but is sometimes more than this with their more objective quality. It is this that I have loosely defined as archetypal, or used relative synonyms such as collective or transpersonal. This appears to be some sort of bedrock on and in which this somewhat fantastic, poetic and mythic material rests.

My contention is that this is the flow or energetic direction this material takes and which we are the recipients of. This approach is inclusive of the reductive, scientific and academic approaches, but includes so much more than them and is fundamentally primary. It also takes the material into a flowing forward direction, rather than a looking back; it is teleological, meaningful, and potentially prophetic: Time is more a function of the soul, it appears. This is the world that the shaman immerses him/herself in, to draw on material that informs his/her community in a spiritual manner. It is what I am attempting here.

Conclusions

And so to... The Charm of Making:

Anall Nathrach,
Urthvas Bethud,
Dochiel Dienve.

The interpretation:

Dragon's breath,
the charm of death and life,
thy omen of making.

In the film *Excalibur* Merlin utters the charm to summon the breath of the Dragon to propel Uther across the ravine that separates him from the Duke of Cornwall's castle, presumably Tintagel, and the object of his desire, the Duke's wife, Ygraine. In the process the Dragon's breath suspends Uther over the abyss and Merlin commands Uther to shapeshift to the appearance of the Duke, so to lie with Ygraine and conceive Arthur. A nice touch is that at the moment of conception the Duke is elsewhere impaled and dying, in his vain and misguided pursuit of Uther. Conception, hence birth, and now death juxtaposed. The Charm seems to encapsulate this act and its consequences, resting it on the inspiration – breath – of the Dragon, and Uther's desire that has evoked it.

This is seemingly the only act that Merlin performs that might be considered magical, although other perspectives of it can be taken. Magic itself can be seen as a kind of supervening term that includes all the more shamanic qualities that have been discussed to date, set in the marginal and soulful space that ritual – however induced – provides. One conclusion that can be drawn from this is that there is no such thing as magic in the literal everyday sense that someone could be turned into a toad, for example, but that altered states of consciousness induce experiences, which when experienced in daily reality can then be seen to alter and change prior perception and its mental consequences, particularly in the view of others. Magic seems to refer to outcome, as much or as well as to the mechanisms that produced it. To magic we will return, and relatively frequently from here on.

In *Excalibur* the Charm now continues as a leitmotif employed on significant occasions, up to and including Merlin's incarceration at the hands of Morgana, Arthur's half-sister, the mother by the latter of the fateful Mordred. It is also used, somewhat significantly at the healing of Lancelot, ironically via the hand of Guinevere, of his self-inflicted guilt-ridden sword wound. The images of the Dragon and reference to it appear regularly in the movie, most significantly through a mist to induce Morgana out of a charmed state to her own death at her son's hands through the instigation of a resurrected, though somewhat ethereal, Merlin.

As I have now moved into the Charm's association to *Excalibur*, this is maybe the point to digress and explore how Boorman and Pallenberg present Merlin a little further. My purpose in doing this, is that I find it an extraordinarily rich portrayal of him and for many reasons. So, how does Merlin look in this representation, and how does it connect with other themes, including my own?

Merlin is a dominating influence, and it is easy to see that it might have been Boorman's original intention to centre the work around him. Nicol Williamson's portrayal is magisterial and in danger of overshadowing the acting of others, who often seem to find it difficult to fit into archetypal shoes the way he has. That he provides a distinct personality to the character is no distraction; it is a relief that the personal is overlaying the mythic and archetypal that then emerges through it.

When I first saw the movie, and with my relatively scant knowledge then of Merlin and the Grail legends, I didn't immediately recognise the portrayal as based primarily on *Le Morte d'Arthur*, thinking it to be more of a compilation. I suspect this was because I was drawn by the imagery and symbolic expressions, deeply Celtic and Irish, as much as the screenplay; and this was mainly by Merlin's expressions. I suspect that the lack of Christian imagery and reference, as well as the Grail hero being Perceval, was significant in how I appreciated it. However, the Grail itself is quite Eucharistic, although in a primarily healing capacity.

Celtic imagery permeates the movie. The dragon is given a central reference and is a point of departure for a lot of the action and connectivity, such as the lightening with Merlin's first teaching of the dragon to Arthur, and then with it striking the latter in the Church after Mordred's birth, conferring on him the divine wound of the Fisher King of Grail legend significance. Two ravens mark Merlin's entrance at Tintagel and are also present at the death of the Duke of Cornwall. Ravens are significant both in Celtic mythology, but also Nordic, where two accompany Odin. This may or may not be an oblique reference to Merlin as Woden.

I am not entirely sure what to make of the feminine imagery and female representations of it; maybe the screenwriters are not either. Morgana is a condensed figure from myth and made very prominent for various reasons, including Helen Mirren's acting capacity and her enigmatic offscreen relationship with Williamson. The Lady of the Lake and hence the whole Faery

Realm is present, though a little underplayed and distant, particularly if connection back to this realm would be considered important to reinforce the Celtic background. However, Boorman does shy away from sexuality and its connection to magic and fate, which is something I will be taking forward: Choice or film-making necessity? Who knows.

The magical and prophetic sequences have been discussed elsewhere throughout this work. These are laid bare when Merlin prophesies, or maybe warns an already smitten Arthur about Guinevere and Lancelot. Later, in response to his question to Merlin, it is of Arthur begetting a son, though he maybe purposefully neglects to give the relevant detail of this. Both exchanges also reinforce his mentor role to the King. The use of the Charm at significant points and its rendering are strong features, and I find it interesting that it is not written out in the screenplay. Also, the latter contains an original version that was subsequently edited, where many other mythic and Celtic features are present. This is available online, so I will take these comments no further here.

Perceval follows in the footsteps of the mythic Welsh Peredur – also mentioned in the Scottish Myrddin story – and is given pride of place in Chrétien de Troyes account of the Grail late in the 12[th]C. This unfinished work spawned numerous so-called continuations, where Perceval becomes Parzival in the interesting version of Wolfram von Eschenbach. Parzival becomes Parsifal in Wagner's *Ring* and it is the orchestral pieces from Wagner's work that forms a lot of the movie's musical score. In the outpouring of continuations in the more strictly Christian Tradition of this brief 12-13[th]C period, Perceval eventually becomes, or shapeshifts to the saintly, pure and virginal Galahad. The Grail becomes a chalice, its connection to both the Last Supper and the Crucifixion is made, and thus its Christian rehabilitation is complete with others, such as by

Malory icing the cake.

This is a very condensed and rather cynical perspective that will be explored in a bit more detail in Part Two. Yet, when contrasted with *Excalibur*, it does indicate how far the story of the Grail – and Merlin dragged along maybe kicking and screaming – has become separated from its origins. Boorman and Pallenberg do a lot to repair this, in a very different way to others like Tolkien, although even he gives a slightly pessimistic perspective of the Pagan Celtic era slipping into the Otherworld, being superseded by Christianity. I beg to differ; hence this account.

After that relevant detour, back to the *Charm of Making*. I like to put the features contained in the Charm into a pattern that have previously been abbreviated to the dualistic death:rebirth that I refer to as the *Great Cycle of Existence*. In a more expanded form, it could read as birth – life – death – rebirth, maybe with sex flowing through, as it touches all of these states: Yes, death included. I call it a cycle, because from the soul perspective this is what existence is. From a rational and non-spiritual viewpoint, it is linear from conception/birth to death, with what happens before and after considered relatively non-existent. But from a spiritual perspective, conception and then subsequently birth into the world is a transition from the transpersonal to the personal, with life ending as death and the transition back.

This is a circle, but it is worth reinforcing that it is cyclic – hence the name Great Cycle of Existence – and even considered as an evolving spiral. As a condensed appreciation of the Charm, I will be referring to the explored elements as the Great Cycle moving forward. It contains the elements of the Charm that move through *Vita* and my own narrative, the dreams in particular. But before moving on to *Vita*, and as well as anticipating Merlin's presence in *Prophecies* that will be discussed afterwards, I would like to focus on the intriguing figure of Lailoken and how he informs the archetypal picture of Merlin.

Interestingly, there exists a text for Lailoken, being the 12thC *Vita Merlini Silvestris,* which is another source of the literary Merlin and possibly related to Geoffrey's unnamed sources. In general, it seems to me the name Myrddin relates to the more Welsh sources, and that Geoffrey has grafted these on to the semi-historical Lailoken for his own reasons and purposes; but there exists enough confusion without any further idle speculation at this time. Instead, it is the description of Lailoken's life that is intriguing, because it reflects the salient points of *Vita,* as well as clarifying some of the difficulties I have encountered there.

The background of the Battle of Arthuret in 573, the trauma and madness are the same, although it is clearly stated that it is madness that endows Lailoken with the gift of prophecy; a very shamanic view. In this account it is the King – more likely a chieftain – Meldred who imprisons Lailoken, releasing him when he recounts the familiar leaf in the Queen's hair prophecy. Although released, the (unnamed) Queen takes revenge by having him ambushed and killed with a triple death by a rustic gang.

Personally, I always found the character of Rhydderch – supposedly victor at Arthuret – to be somewhat implausible in Geoffrey's *Vita;* being alternatively relatively weak (at least at court) and ambivalent with regard to Merlin. I also find it odd that his Queen, when unmasked as an adulteress, nonetheless becomes Merlin's close ally in the forest. However, at least here there is clarification of a more substantial Meldred, although the similarity to Maeldin in *Vita* and others, such as Mordred, continue to raise questions for me. Here the Queen acts more plausibly and demonstrates her own – quite Celtic – strength and possible independence. Unlike Gwenddydd with Merlin, she has no relationship to Lailoken; unless, of course, he was the lover and therefore this not a prophecy, but a ruse to obtain his release. Also, the triple death is not a prophecy but more an execution. As an aside, the Queen's infidelity does resonate with the behaviour of Arthur's wife and the broader issue of fidelity and sexuality in Celtic thought: More to come here.

This raises various questions for me. The role of Gwendolen strikes me as being somewhat peripheral, and her new husband's death part of something more shamanic and even initiatory; maybe it is an interjected story, rather like the beggar prophecy, which then shores up the prophetic stock to support Geoffrey's view of Merlin. By contrast, Gwenddydd is more substantial, rather like Meldred's wife, although I consider her not to be Merlin's sister; I suspect this is Geoffrey simply doing further sanitary work with regard to the Church. I believe she is his lover and/or *soror mystica*, and maybe the forerunner of the enchantress and Merlin's enigmatic and supposed death by entombment that I will come to, although in *Vita* any supposed entrapment is voluntary and relative.

Gwenddydd's name means 'The Dawn' and indicates a symbolic level, as there is with Lailoken that means 'Wise Fool'. Although the latter is certainly descriptive, it reminds me of the Fool in the Tarot, which points to Tarot imagery elsewhere in these various accounts. The Dawn may indicate Gwenddydd's role as an awakener, and potentially a sexual one. This reinforces the 'seductive enchantress' image of Merlin's younger consort in later accounts. Sex and power come together, again. It seems Geoffrey has symbolised and even romantisised a lot of the core material around Merlin, basing it more on Lailoken than the other various sources for Merlin. Not that this has been forgotten, as Myrddin makes significant interjections in his account, even if indirect. But for the more fundamental and

Welsh view of Merlin, *Prophecies* will be looked at in more detail, where the alchemical themes of the elements, in particular water in the triple death and the healing spring, will be examined further.

Overall, *Vita* has all the qualities of a syncretic work informed by many sources focused around the life or lives of a figure or figures who lived in the late 6thC in the Scottish Lowlands. It seems Geoffrey was trying to unify these figures for the various reasons already raised, and because these stories were obviously still current, mainly in folk form, although now being increasingly subjected to literature. It seems Geoffrey wanted to have his say and retain the connection to Welsh sources around Myrddin, in particular, but also to connect these all back to the Merlin he had given birth to in *Prophecies* and the relatively more historical accounts in oral tradition.

What I have tried to do is link this story, as well as the ones immediately surrounding it, to the background tradition of shamanism and the core archetypal process provided in the Great Cycle of Existence. That trauma, grief and madness is rife conforms to shamanic tradition particularly, but it also links to the Great Cycle via death and ultimately Merlin's own, if the triple death is re-read as in Lailoken's story. Prophecy is a major theme that Geoffrey brings to the fore, magic only indirectly. Various themes of sex and power are evident, even if only as undercurrents, healing being more apparent and direct. Sex points to the ensuing bête noir of the Church, and is relatively understated, though will become more apparent as I step further into the feminine world in Part Two. That I refer to disciplines such as alchemy is because I can and will further see the relevance of the associated runes to this account, but also because alchemy is a direct descendent of shamanism, particular from the Iron Age onward; it is also a close cousin of magic, maybe even more so than prophecy.

There are some significant conclusions to my mind, such as the resonance of various patterns – the Queen's infidelity for one – to the Arthurian legends that *Vita* and other works were spawned by and furthered. But more intriguing is the relationship of this material to Nordic mythology and the figure of Odin, via the somewhat transitional yet autonomous Anglo-Saxon Woden, who I see as a forerunner of Merlin. This association with Nordic mythology is present not only in Lailoken's name, but the significant triple death and additional features, like the ash tree. These also link not only to elemental alchemy, but also and inevitably back to shamanism. More issues could be brought in, such as the significance of laughter in mania and shamanism; the various bindings that Merlin receives at Rhydderch's hands; the reason why Geoffrey introduced the killing of Gwendolen's husband; the stag and its horns as symbols; and even the role of Gwendolen herself. Some of these will return as I progress, yet there seems more than enough already to build on. But before progressing to *Prophecies*, I would like to link this material back to my own narrative.

At first blush, there does not appear to be much of significance in the Childhood Dream beyond symbolic trauma of varied origins. Yet, when I expand upon it and bring in associations, there is more than first meets the eye. This is mostly around the Great Cycle, with sex and death. Sex is implied in the phallic nature of the pylon shape; although a little vague, it becomes reinforced by the fountain in the Original Dream and further in a dream yet to come. Sex is also there by association with my father and his lover's site of trysting. This is directly associated with power; not only the inherent power of the pylon, but its power over me.

Yet there is also what is absent in the dream that is notable. My sister's trauma is significant because of my solitude in the walk. It is a journey with initiatory overtones, as my – maybe interim – intention is set by its repetitious insistence on being heard. The dark-brooding of my rejected and unavailable mother hangs over the dream, a connection I am not and never do re-establish at that level; that is mine to deal with in other ways. Yet there is more: It is prophetic in a manner that will reveal itself in other dreams – as recounted here – and over time; it is initiatory; it has levels of association and connection that will occur and recur; and it is potentially transformative, in that I am directed away from a regressive solution in a relatively dysfunctional family setting.

The Original Dream expands on some of this. Most notably is the pylon related to the metallic fountain sculpture with the cut-off top, which is more distinctly phallic (and where most of my attention was located at the time of dreaming). Yet this is not only sexual, erotic and powerful, it is also leading me into something deeper – the Grail-like jewel: My sexuality was, at this time, something to go through and transform. The healing nature of the fountain, as with the healing spring of Merlin's madness in the forest, indicates the centrality of this psychic dynamic and locates it with the water element, as with Merlin, and reinforced by the image of the Pacific Ocean.

Yet the nature and history of Hiroshima hangs over the dream like a death pall, paradoxically associated with the birth of a new island: A transformation. The tension of the opposites – Pacific:Hiroshima – is crucial; somehow the tension must be maintained for the healing to emerge. Trauma is not to be foregone, but weathered, sustained, even *remembered*. There will be more to say about these features in Part Two, which resonates with the first half of this dream, yet also links to what has been discussed to date.

In the countryside I am the doctor, my career at the time. Julie is a kind of alchemical soror mystica, erotic more than sexual, and is my link to my patients and work. The various women provide this function in *Vita*, with Gwenddydd ultimately 'succeeding' Merlin in the prophetic arts and joining with him in the inner core of his entourage. I sense this is prophetic for me, as well; once the demands and intentions of this dream are fulfilled – which this work is doing – it is a realm I may well also pass into.

I feel I am still wrestling with the pattern of the original man, woman and their son, even though it is the man on whom my attention becomes focused. There are almost Freudian connotations here, particularly if the sexual and traumatic factors dotted throughout this account are considered, yet I am more inclined to see the religious overtones here as a feminine Trinity, of sorts. I will be wrestling further with this in Part Two, but for now my attention is on the man. Although *original* can mean something that is created directly or unique, here I incline to seeing it in the sense of primal, fundamental... even archetypal.

The mists are of the Dragon, its breath or even inspiration and representing the veil between the worlds. Is the man an ancestor, as in the alternative rendering of the charm as *come hither ye* ancestors? Who am I, in relation to the man? I am not his son; I am his healer. He is tired, worn out, rather like Arthur in *Excalibur* before he is revived by drinking from the Grail that Perceval has retrieved. Is what is in the jar what I will need a vice to open? I suspect it is, because it is directly related to my being a doctor and using this to probably heal him. But I'll need a vice to open it.

Is the man Arthur and am I Perceval? I had thought not, but I am beginning to reconsider... He is not dressed as a King, he looks more like a priest in casual, yet smart clothing. It is my conviction that he is, of course, at one level myself; in that I am now – over 40 years later – like he and have been, or still am in need of rejuvenation or process of transition, spiritual rather than physical. There is a dream to come that will clarify him further, but, in the meantime, I contend that he and I are somehow wrestling with Merlin and his rejuvenation into an era that is in need of him; if not, why would a figure like Gandalf so capture the collective imagination?

The jar itself will make a deeper connection to Merlin and dragons in the forthcoming *Prophecies* section; it also has alchemical connotations. The word vice has intrigued me for many a year. It would seem practical, as in a vice to grip and open the jar by means of its mechanical power, but is it more. Vice also means immoral or even criminal. There are Faustian undertones here... Immorality implies – for me – nefarious sexuality, possibly drink and drugs; criminality doesn't ring any bells. Sex and power, sex and shamanism (drugs), the drugs of my healing trade as a doctor. It is the power aspect I most feel here, with the potential to walk the path of individuation rather than one bounded by expectation and duty. Maybe there is more to unravel... on to *Prophecies* in the meantime.

Prophecies

The Mythic Background

What follows is an updated and rather sanitised version of the classic myth centred around Merlin and Vortigern, taken from Richard Barber, *Myths and Legends of the British Isles*:

> *At last he (Vortigern) took the advice of his wizards, who told him that he ought to build an exceedingly strong tower, since he had lost all his other castles. He searched everywhere to find a suitable place, and at last came to Snowdon. Here he assembled a great gang of masons from various countries, and ordered them to build the tower. The stonemasons began to lay the foundations, but whatever they did one day was swallowed up by the earth the next, so they did not know where their work had disappeared to. Vortigern, when he heard about this, once more asked his wizards to tell him the reason for this. They said that he must search for a boy who had never had a father; and when he had found him, he should kill him and sprinkle his blood over the mortar and the stones. This, they said, would make the foundation of the tower hold firm.*
>
> *Messengers were sent everywhere to look for such a boy. When they came to Carmarthen, they saw some lads playing before the gate: they sat down, weary with*

travel, and looked round them in the hope of finding what they sought. Towards evening, a couple of youths whose names were Merlin and Dalbutius suddenly quarrelled; and as they argued, Dalbutius said to Merlin: 'What a fool you are to think you are a match for me! I come from royal blood on both my mother's and father's side, but no one knows who you are, because you never had a father!' At this the messengers pricked up their ears, and asked the bystanders who this Merlin might be. They told them that no one knew his father, but that his mother was daughter of the king of Dyfed, and that she lived with the nuns in St Peter's Church in that same city.

The messengers hurried off to the reeve of the city, and ordered him in the king's name to have Merlin and his mother sent to the king. When he learnt of their errand, the reeve at once sent Merlin and his mother to Vortigern for him to do whatever he wanted with them. And when they were brought into his presence, the king received the mother with due respect knowing that she was of noble birth. Then he asked her who the father of her son might be.

She replied: 'On my soul, my lord king, I know of no man who was his father. All I can tell you is that once, when I and my attendants were in our chambers, someone appeared to me in the shape of a handsome young man, who embraced me and kissed me and stayed with me for some time. Then he suddenly vanished and I never saw him again: he often spoke to me when I was alone, though I never saw him. When he had haunted me in this way for a long time I conceived and bore a child. This is the truth, my lord king, whatever you may make of it; I know of no one who is the father of this boy.'

Amazed by her words, the king asked for Maugantius to be brought; and when the latter had heard the story from first to last, he said to Vortigern: 'In books and histories written by wise men I have found that many men have been born in this way. Apuleius says that there are certain spirits between the moon and the earth, which we call incubi. Their nature is partly human, partly angelic, and they take on the shape of men at will and associate with mortal women. Perhaps one of these appeared to this lady and is the father of the youth.'

When Merlin heard all this, he came to the king and said: 'Why have my mother and I been summoned here?'

Vortigern answered: 'My wizards have declared that I should seek out a boy who never had a father, because when I have sprinkled his blood upon the foundation of the tower I am building it will stand firm.'

Merlin said: 'Summon your wizards and I will show that they are lying.'

The king, amazed at his words, summoned his wizards so that Merlin could confront them. Merlin said to them: 'Don't you know what is preventing the foundation of this tower from being laid? You have advised that it should be built with mortar mixed with my blood, to make it stand securely. But ask yourselves what is hidden under the foundation, which prevents it from standing?' The wizards were frightened and said nothing.

Then Merlin (who was also called Ambrosius) said: 'My lord king, call your workmen and get them to dig, and you will find a pool under the tower that prevents it from standing.'

They did this, and a pool was indeed discovered.

Then Merlin Ambrosius again questioned the wizards: 'Tell me now, you liars and flatterers, what is under the pool?' But they were all dumb and said not a word. He said to the king: 'Order that the pool is to be drained; in the bottom you will find two dragons asleep.' The king did so, since Merlin had been proved right about the pool; and once more, to his astonishment, he found that it was as Merlin said. And after that, Merlin prophesied the future history of Britain, to the amazement and bafflement of his hearers.

When Vortigern had listened to him, he wanted to learn what his own fate would be; and Merlin's answer was as follows:

'Escape from the fire of the sons of Constantine, if you can! At this very moment they are fitting out their ships; at this very moment they are leaving the coast of Brittany and sailing out into the open sea towards Britain, which they will invade. They will defeat the accursed Saxons, but before that they will besiege you in a tower and set fire to it. It was your actions that brought this fate upon you when you betrayed their father and invited the Saxons into Britain as your bodyguard; they will come over as your executioners. Two deaths await you, and I cannot tell which of them you will escape. The Saxons will lay waste your kingdom and will try to kill you. And Aurelius and Uther Pendragon will invade your lands seeking revenge for their father's death. So take refuge if you can. Tomorrow they will land at Totnes. The Saxons

128

will suffer bloody injuries: Hengist will be killed, and
Aurelius Ambrosius will be crowned king. He will
reign in peace and will restore the churches, but he will
die of poison. His brother Uther Pendragon will
succeed him, but his reign will also be cut short by
poison. Your descendants will be there when this
happens, and Uther's son Arthur will revenge his
father!'

As an aside: A little earlier I pointed to Tarot symbolism in *Vita*, specifically the Fool card. Also, regarding Merlin, the Hanged Man card could be appropriate, as well as the Magician. Here, somewhat obviously to those familiar, is the Tower of Destruction. The purpose of mentioning this is not to try and specifically ally the Tarot with the mythic structure here, but to point out its scattered imaginative emergence, thus indicating the profound depth and archetypal presence in these various accounts and the Tarot.

The above is one of many accounts that could have been shared regarding this story, as it is written more as history, rather than from the Celtic myths from which it originates. I have used it, because in our era it is the one that is most recognisable. To my appreciation it seems constructed chronologically later and for reasons apart from the embedded historicisation. The most obvious is the Christianisation of the tale, which I won't go into any further here, as there has been comment already and there will also be more appreciation of this process in Part Two; by now it must be obvious how the process of recorded history has glossed the Pagan and Celtic tales that are deeply embedded here.

Named Merlin, although with reference to Ambrosius, thus following Nennius in his Romanesque naming, it therefore postdates Geoffrey. In fact, this tale is quite weighted toward the Roman-British connection as with the various names. Other accounts are more traditional, and include the boy as the Welsh Emrys. Naming Merlin as Ambrosius, which then recurs as the king Aurelius Ambrosius, is unexplained and more than a little intriguing. Aurelius is Uther's brother and hence Arthur's uncle; uncles have a significant mentor role in older cultures... There is possibly more to this story than meets the eye at first glance, given that Ambrose can be white or blue as a colour – think alchemy here – and represent the feminine; as a name it could mean *immortal.*

More significant to me and this present study is that there are "two dragons asleep" at the bottom of the pool, whereas in other accounts these dragons are encased in eggs or vases (see later). They emerge from these, one red and one white, and ascend fighting each other. Initially the white dragon was favoured, though ultimately the red was the victor. Merlin interprets this as the white being the Saxons and the red the indigenous British, who ultimately triumph. Interestingly, there are resonances of this in the rivalry of the War of the Roses in medieval times, indicating a currency to the accounts that contain this symbolism. Although the water is preserved as the pool (and also as the feminine), this may relate to the actual historical story of a failure to build such a castle in Snowdonia at Dinas Emrys, because of its watery nature.

There is deep symbolism of an alchemical nature here that is being excluded at the expense of Merlin's prophetic utterances about Vortigern's future and the arrival of Arthur, thus forging the connection for time immemorial. This symbolism can also be seen as sexual, particularly to those of a spiritually eastern inclination, which – to me – resonates with Merlin's unnamed mother and her relationship to his unknown father; this lack of naming being all the more significant when others, including the seemingly peripheral Dalbutius, are named with their Roman significance. That there is also a distinct resonance here with the

Greek Eros-Psyche myth should not be overlooked, in spite of the Christianisation and demonisation of Merlin's father as an incubus. Also, given the earlier explanation of my own spiritual name, is that the description of Merlin's father readily fits an elf.

After the simple finding of the dragons, "Merlin prophesied the future history of Britain" starting with Vortigern. Yet, hidden behind this simple statement are Geoffrey's *Prophecies*, radically excluded in this account. These may have been penned by Geoffrey and the product of his own fevered imagination, but they are nevertheless quite prophetic. They are almost inaccessible to the modern mentality and it would take me too far afield to include them here, as they lend themselves to independent exploration. It interests me that we have explored prophetic utterances of people like Nostradamus, yet in our own traditional Celtic backyard is a collection of prophecies of an otherworldly and initiatory nature that we have not explored or connected to.

To substantiate some of my prior comments, here is the relevant part of another relatively historical account (Michael Senior, *Myths of Britain*):

> *Messengers, the Nennius story continues, were sent out. In the south of Wales they found a boy who claimed to have no father, and they brought him north to Snowdon. Confronted on the hilltop with his imminent death, he demanded to question the wise men. What was it, he asked, that was hidden under the paving on the hill's summit? They did not know, but he did. There was a pool there. They opened the paving, and found the pool. And what was in the pool? he asked. To their ignorance he replied that there were two containers; on separating the containers they would find a wrapping — literally a 'tent' between*

two 'vases'; and in the wrapping two serpents, one of them white, the other red. All this was discovered as predicted, and when they then unfolded the cloth and released the serpents he told them also what would happen next. The serpents began to fight each other, the white one at first winning, and then, after the third near defeat, the red one recovering and finally driving out the white. The king and his magicians stood astonished as the prophetic boy explained all this to them. The pool, he told them, was the world, the tent Vortigern's kingdom. The two serpents were the dragons of two nations, the red one that of the natives of Britain, the white one the invading Saxons. In the end, he said, our people will drive out the Saxons and send them back to where they came from. But as far as Vortigern was concerned, there was no future for him on this hill. It was he, the boy, who should have control of the castle to be built there. He gave his name then: Ambros.

When I approached this section, I had anticipated using Geoffrey's *Prophecies* to continue the earlier theme around *Vita*. But I experienced a writing resistance and for weeks chose not to continue, needing to listen to what was behind the resistance, I surmised. Then I had a dream that told me to get on with the account, but to rely more on my own understanding of prophecies and prophesying, rather than to take recourse to Geoffrey. I felt I had seen enough of him: Although his place in the Merlin story is significant, even pivotal, I was increasingly drawn to the mythic material from which he drew inspiration, and I had the Grail – prefaced in my Original Dream – yet to contend with. And Geoffrey had not furthered this direction, though others did and some with the literary and hence mythic use and furtherance of Merlin's involvement, which intrigued me.

Yet I do not want to get too drawn into the interpretation of the myths in which these stories are embedded, because that would reduce them too much to our daily perception and consciousness. Instead, I want to look at the mythic content in its more *Otherworldly* context. By this, I am referring to what others may refer to as the *collective unconscious* (Jung) or the *supersensible reality* (Rudolf Steiner and others) with the term *Otherworld*. Even history can be seen to unfold from this, as is relatively obvious here, when the material is taken from the mythic and pre-historical background of the British or Celtic peoples and interpreted in a historical manner to justify personal ambitions; more politics than prophecy at play in that case though, I would suggest.

Prophecy stems from this otherworldly reality, that is (relatively) beyond space and time, self-regulating, autonomous and of immense power: Recall the omnipotent, omniscient and omnipresent triad that defines 'God' as well as the characteristics of Jungian archetypes? Myth is an expression of this reality in artistic form, principally musically and poetically in those times. To enter this virtual space means crossing a threshold into a marginal or liminal reality, using ritual practice as conducted by those with a more shamanic sensibility, or by other appropriate tools. Here, the visionary experience is prophetic and stands outside of time and space. It is paradoxical and enigmatic by its very nature, and only predictive when it is brought back into daily reality and interpreted in this context.

Prophecy stands in its own right and, at a deep level, remains resistant to rational interpretation. That Geoffrey placed Merlin here, as an alternative to Ambrose or even Emrys, is not mythically incompatible with the more historically based account of him later in the sixth century, associated with other names and in a different location. This earlier Merlin is a child prophet, itself a mythic identity, born of a union that resonates with the Jesus story and that of many other similar figures in myth and sometimes associated with historical figures: Maybe it was Geoffrey's intent to juxtapose the two?

With this understanding, it will be of ongoing value to distil the core symbolism and give it some sort of significance and interpretation, notwithstanding my preceding comments on this point. Interestingly, whilst we commonly see the image of the serpent as relatively synonymous with the dragon, here the "two serpents were the dragons of two nations". Whilst this statement implies equivalence, there is also a sense that the dragon is more symbolic or totemic, which as a mythic creature it is in contrast to the serpent that is a large snake, commonly associated with treachery and specifically the devil in Christianity. Maybe the dragon predates or has escaped the Christian clutches here? Apart from their mythic nature, the significant difference is that the dragon breaths out fire, which is of elemental and alchemical significance. The first stage of alchemy is calcination where the element of fire is used to initiate the transformative process.

In the story, and although described as 'vases', the containers sound more like eggs with the tent or wrapping as the membranous covering of the womb that holds the growing being; alternatively, a vase in alchemy – called an *athanor* – could be the container in which the transformative process occurs. Separation is a culinary term, but also signifies the stage in alchemy following dissolution that is watery, and hence the pond.

The fourth stage of alchemy is conjunction, the unification of the white and red. Initially the white dragon predominates, which also signifies the end of this phase of alchemy, known as the Lesser Work. Then follows the Greater Work through putrefaction, fermentation, distillation and finally coagulation.

This is marked by the colour red and is the highest stage of enlightenment. In essence, this story as a prophetic utterance from Merlin sounds more like an alchemical formula than a genuine prediction, so may represent the continuation of tradition in a disguised form. There is a deep and rather obscure tradition of Druid Alchemists, sometimes referred to as *Pheryllt* or *Fferyllt*; I vaguely wonder whether Merlin is a representative of or a practitioner in this tradition, as much or even more than being a Druid.

From a more sexual perspective, the eggs could be the ovaries or the testicles, or even the two developing foetuses in the womb. Irrespective, this indicates fertility and – in and of itself – growth and transformation. In some spiritual traditions, the red and white represent two channels that entwine the central one in the spine; sexual excitement is then initiated to awaken these energies and foster their ascent and union to the symbolic crown above the head. There are gender implications here, as the white is the more active component that rises to the more passive and male red, a distinct pattern in eastern spiritual systems. The parallels across broader cultures here are intriguing and potentially informative of the deep level, maybe historically and mythologically, from which this present story may have emerged.

Whilst this story is used here in a more political manner; that is, interpreted into a prediction of the time with the Saxons and Britons, it has a continuation into the medieval era of the ensuing millennium. It becomes used as a political tool to justify the actions of those seeking power and control of the land. The house of Plantagenet ruled from 1154, when Henry II was crowned after Stephen, to 1485 when the Tudor dynasty began following the ascension of the House of Lancaster, as symbolised by the red rose (the white rose being the House of York): Further levels of prophesy? These varied interpretations and tenuous relationship of prediction to prophecy are marked over time. So, the question would be: Is this prophecy still playing out and, if it is, what significance does it have in our era?

Prophecy and The Charm

Maybe one area of this significance is the creation of the above charm by the writers of *Excalibur*, prophecy as magic, maybe?

> *Dragon's breath,*
> *the charm of death and life,*
> *thy omen of making.*

Before starting, here is a sketch of the meaning of the various words that have become unfamiliar or even debased in our time. A *charm* is a magical act, including a *spell* or the use of words; it also has a magical association embraced in modern usage, as in the term *charming*. As an object of magical power, it is known as a *talisman* or *amulet*; although somewhat equivalent, the word amulet is of Latin derivation and is considered more protective in nature. *Omen* is regarded as a portent of good or evil, even carrying *prophetic significance*; it also indirectly illustrates the relationship between prophecy and prediction outlined earlier.

Whilst the Charm overlaps the comments about alchemy, above, it has much more of a direct magical quality about it, as indicated by the wording itself. Magic is a somewhat ephemeral term, subject to varying definition by differing commentators and practitioners. Some of my own observations and deductions in this regard follow.

I consider *magic* to be almost a supervening term for the various ones above; that is, charm, spell, omen and the like. It is possibly better described than defined, although its association to disciplines such as alchemy are a help. If prophecy is magical, it indicates that magic is the ability to step into a different order of reality, probably through such states as altered ones of consciousness, immersion in art, creativity, hallucinogenic drugs, fasting, sleep deprivation, sexuality etc. This reality I have described as the collective unconscious of Jung, or the supersensible reality of Steiner and others; there are many such descriptions, depending on which framework is being used.

What does seem to be important is the use of ritual to enter into this space through an in-between or intermediate state called *liminality*. Without the inherent protection of psychic boundaries provided by ritual, one flirts with insanity, not frenzied madness and genuine ecstasy. This liminal state is wherein everyday consciousness and rationality in particular, are suspended. Here, a passive and receptive position can be undertaken, as with the art of divination, or an act of creation. Magic is when one specifically enters into the hypothetical *space* beyond conventional space and time in a visionary (considered both image and sound; visual and auditory) capacity, and there interacts with it and any apparent beings encountered. What emanates from this place and brought back can be prophetic, in the form of words, and magical, with relevant acts; often in combination. It can also be vehicle of healing, inasmuch as magic can be employed in this capacity.

The Charm could be considered both prophetic and magical, depending on how it is used and as portrayed in *Excalibur*. It is magical when used at the beginning to summon the Dragon's breath so that a transformed Uther can lie with Ygraine. It is also magical when Morgana uses it to entrap Merlin, but then in an interesting inversion similarly portends her death later. It is used for healing when Lancelot is wounded, and with Guinevere's assistance, indicating a shamanic element. It is prophetic in that it induces altered states of consciousness or liminality in the stone circle, as an otherworld portal maybe, and generally elsewhere.

The specifics of the Charm are in the poetic wording. The breath of the dragon produces a mist or fog in the movie, probably in expiration. What is intriguing is that the elements of air, as in inspiration, and fire are juxtaposed. They are so in alchemy, as well as being masculine from a gender perspective. It is as if there is an appeal to the beyond, the world of *spirit*. The charm wording, as a *spell*, juxtaposes death and life, as earlier indicated in the movie when the Duke of Cornwall dies at the same time that Arthur is conceived. In fact, I prefer the word spell here instead of charm in line 2, negating any obfuscation with the actual name of the Charm itself, which also points to a broader meaning of charm in contrast to spell.

The Charm is also present in Merlin's entrapment, and subsequently with the bewitchment when it is used by Merlin – in an altered state of consciousness – to dispossess Morgana of her magical appearance and propel her towards her death, ironically at the hands of her son. It may be worth mentioning that in French, sexual orgasm is connoted as *le petit mort*, or the *little death* that prefaces an altered state of consciousness.

Omen is the outcome of the lines that precede it, the portent of the prophecy. Consequently, there is a *making*; in the context of the movie this is Arthur's conception, but can also be seen more broadly as change, transition or transformation. This is the case whenever the Charm is used in the movie; it marks something significant, alerting those involved (including we, as the audience) that something different and important is going to happen; in other words, it is magic in action.

Myth, Dream and Prophecy

Components that augment prophecy include healing, sacrifice and initiation. This is readily apparent in the Jesus myth, one that has dominated our time and tended to exclude others, particularly those of our own tradition and background. The figures of Woden and Merlin, along with their shamanic attributes, stand tall in this with their relative similarities and revivification in our time, as Christianity loses its religious grip on our religious worldview with the resurgence of Pagan and indigenous spiritual traditions worldwide. It is the end of an era.

It is common to look to dreams for answers to everyday problems or to make predictions into the future. These are dim remembrances of the deeper functioning of the dreaming process that is more prophetic in nature; although, of course, most common dreaming does not reach to these collective levels, but provides a kind of complementary feedback in the form of information. As an aside: Nor are or should dreams be used as solutions to daily problems; our obligation is to *listen* to and *watch* the symbolic and metaphoric data to compensate for an incomplete or imbalanced conscious daily attitude.

So-called *Big Dreams* (a term borrowed from Amerindian traditions) have a more holistic effect, in that we are affected mentally, emotionally and physically by them, in various combinations; they are potentially transformative. The extension to this is that such dreams are ultimately spiritual in origin, providing us not only with information, but also meaning, direction and purpose. Such dreams occur to the individual, but many cultures see them as having a wider social importance and they can be shared in a communal space, as they are deemed relevant to the people or tribe as a whole.

The Childhood Dream was repetitive in nature, demanding to be heard beyond my fear. When I finally faced it – in the dream context – I was able to stop its incessant calling; I had started to listen. However, I did not understand it at the time, it is only much later that this has begun to occur. It was prophetic in that it provided a depth and context for what was happening as an undercurrent in my life and later I could see predictive elements in it, particularly when I connected the symbolic imagery to other dreams; most specifically the Original Dream here, and one I have yet to come to. It was an initiation into a different phase of my life, a sacrifice of the idyllic past that actually never was, and healing in that, I came to accept the limitations of my upbringing and my parents' hidden behaviour.

The pylon image made little sense to me at the time, and it was with the Original Dream that I could relate it to the sculpture in the fountain. Although this imagery has been explored, there is more to come; but I have assigned this first part of the dream to Part Two of this work, so will leave this exegesis at this point until then, when the Sacrificial Dream is also portrayed and explored.

In the second half of the Original Dream, I have nominated a Merlinesque quality and context to the figures there, even though there are various others that could be used. The mists, their Celtic flavour, and resonance with the Charm reinforce this assessment. Indeed, it is relevant to do this; to explore the various pathways that open up, such as the Trinitarian and Freudian ones, to see where they go and how they impact on the whole picture that emerges. I realise now it had a prophetic quality, even though I did not appreciate it in this way at that time. It had a deep emotional impact and has stayed present within me, even drawing me into this present work.

The male figure at the end of the dream is older and worn out; even at the time I had a sense this was talking about – predicting – my future. Because I now see myself this way, and the garb to indicate both a religious and a philosophical disposition, although in a modern context. He is in need of healing and at the time – I was present and active in this doctor role after all – I had and still have the necessary tools to do this. Interestingly, these are not medical but more shamanic; the jar recalls the vases of the dragons beneath Vortigern's failed tower. Did and does this relate to the undercurrents of the man's malaise?

Shamanistically, I am the healer, a role I have foregone in any formal medical capacity, but present still in other contexts. The vice indicates – to me – power and also sexuality, but in a condensed form and maybe yet to reveal itself fully. We tend to separate these two qualities and give negative connotations to them, particularly with sexuality as a vice; I contend this is a fundamental dualistic error. Yet sexuality has been a significant undercurrent of my life, even to authorship of two associated books. Sex permeates the dream, even if indirectly, as it does the others under examination here. Sex and power are admixed in Merlin's image, as the older man supposedly besotted with a younger woman or muse, who retains her favours and uses their power to entrap him. Am I liberating him, with my healing abilities, from this now redundant and Christianised image?

The tales of Merlin in and around *Vita* paint a different and contrasting picture. In Geoffrey he is vaguely associated with sex, recognising his sister's infidelity, but otherwise he has a sexually sanitised image to become part of an almost monastic collective of people at the end of his life, although maybe this is written from Geoffrey's clerical perspective. In contrast, the more wretched Lailoken undergoes the triple death. It seems the image of Merlin as the besotted pensioner is a relatively later and more Christian one. But does this represent entrapment or a voluntary withdrawal; temporary (as in 'retreat' or attaining visions in a liminal space) or permanent; facilitated by the female companion as muse or soror mystica? Is this what Julie signifies in the Original Dream?

What can be gleaned from these intersecting alternatives is that when prophecy enters the daily world it attracts all sorts of accretions from the people that relate to it with their vested interests. Most notable in this study is the Christian Church, with the movement away from oral and poetic expression to the written word. Pagan traditions value the spoken word more highly, with its mythic expression in ritual, ceremony and theatre; unless poetically employed, maybe the written word represents an abstraction or devaluation in contexts such as these.

But, of course, I have my accretions too. What I am attempting to do is identify them and strip them away from the core mythic and archetypal material that stands behind or beneath these significant, or big dreams. This is soul territory, where myth can be heard directly and free of such accretions and other encumbrances. It is moving from daily reality to a liminal space, where this revealed material can be witnessed and experienced directly. This is something that the Church has limited, by demonising the Pagan perspective, reducing the soul to its partial expression in the afterlife, and acting as an interpretative go-between from spirit to man, as in the Eucharist. There is a level of irony here, when the Grail is considered as the cup of the Last Supper.

Merlin and Prophecy

There are glimpses of the prophetic and predictive in *Excalibur*, although this is almost as enigmatic to define and describe in any detail as magic itself, with which by now it must be evident that there is an overlapping and intimate relationship. Both deal with the Otherworld (a Celtic term), the collective unconscious, spiritual reality or whatever term suits one's disposition. What is interesting is that both the Otherworld and Jung's collective unconscious posit a feminine portal, usually in the form of a woman as muse, soror mystica, anima etc. There are other feminine attributes, such as elemental water, which support this overall perspective. Some, including me, associate these attributes to the soul and hence this being the portal, accessed in liminal space, that communicates with the world of spirit as well as by entering into it, like the shaman.

Merlin's relationship with the wily Morgana is a latter-day picture of the mage. Drawn from Malory's *Le Morte d'Arthur* it marks the close of his journey through medieval literature and by this point is well Christianised. The feminine is demonised, hence making her relatively inaccessible to the ensuing modern mentality, except in the hands of poets and artists. Unfortunately, the mud has stuck, and one has to go back to well before Geoffrey to gain a more balanced perspective. This is in Celtic myth, which is drawn upon by the likes of Nennius and Geoffrey, and reaches a heightened and esoterically mature form in the ensuing Grail legends.

What I believe is true is that the movie indicates the dynamic of Merlin's entrapment as one of power, and is not primarily sexual. The authenticity of this statement is that Merlin is "not a man" and sexuality not a portal of seduction; he is, effectively, more than a little beyond the Great Cycle already. Later interpretations of the myth around sexuality are an attempt to paint it darkly and invoke repression in the listener; somewhat ironic that the Church would use its power in this way, methinks.

Specifically, Merlin's relationship with his sister Gwenddydd, or Ganieda, strikes me as odd, unless 'sister' is seen as a euphemism for lover (as in: Was Merlin the lover who rolled in the grass in her husband Rhydderch's castle?) and, in his later life a prophetess in her own right, as well as a soror mystica to Merlin prior. The relationship of significance in his prophetic youth is Merlin's mother who, interestingly, is unnamed, although considered from regal background. All these seem hints or indirect references to a significant female figure, one who is replete in Celtic culture, even to the point of being synonymous with the divine. I suspect this goes too far, as my dream seems to indicate, but it is certainly a more balanced view than that of modernity, even if she is given a psychological interpretation as Merlin's feminine nature or soul image.

Yet, tantalisingly, there is a specific body of work called *Prophecies* that was Geoffrey's first work, later to be included in his *History*. This was not an afterthought, but the recognition that at this time myth, history and prophecy were intimately connected. It is not my intention to relate or go into any content detail of the actual prophecies, except to remark that they are obscure (even more so than Nostradamus' quatrains), astrological, with classical features that, rather like *Vita*, indicate that they were a product of Geoffrey's inspired imagination. This does not invalidate them, particularly as at that time authorship was often attributed elsewhere, but indicates that, in this period at least, prophetic insight was highly valued. For its time, *Prophecies* was an outstanding literary success, particularly when integrated with *History*.

The *Prophecies* may have had a more immediate function, relating to the political events of the time. But one feature of genuine prophecy is that it is many-levelled; coming as it does from a timeless reality, it can be seen to intersect at various points in timebound history. Given that this was at a historical time when these levels of reality were considered closer than today and even overlapping; there was thus not the same need or desire to separate history from myth and prophecy. Indeed, they were seen as bound together. It is only our modern sensibility that has separated and disconnected them, such that we live in a metaphoric two-dimensional flatland that lacks depth and access to multi-dimensionality.

In this likewise manner, it was not uncommon to link genealogies to significant mythic figures, even considered gods by some. This is true of the Anglo-Saxon shamanic god Woden (Odin in Scandinavia), although in later times after the Conquest at the turn of the millennium it was Arthur who gained more prominence. In my opinion, Arthur is primarily a mythic figure of archetypal import to and for the future Kings of Britain. Of course, his significance cannot now be viewed without reference to Merlin, which I bring into question, certainly in degree.

Woden is an interesting figure in this study. *Wod* (or *Od* in Old Norse) means inspiration, usually of the poetic kind, although I am reminded of the Charm and the *Dragon's breath*. *Den/Din* may relate to a god-man, as is also present with *Myrddin*. What is interesting here is that the prefix *Myr* does not relate to inspiration, or the element air, but water: How feminine and Celtic. Merlin certainly has a strong relationship to water, not only with Vortigern's tower, but in the various *Lady of the Lake* identities that crop up in the myths. What I am suggesting here is an overlap, as there is even a Welsh god and magician called *Gwyddion*. This is all very suggestive and indicates some sort of archetypal unity and associated prophetic function.

Take a step across the North Sea – regularly traversed in pre-Christian times (the Anglo-Saxon 'invasions' were nothing new) – and we find Odin as the most significant mythic figure of the time in question. Odin is considered to have an ambiguous sexuality relating both to the magic called *galdr*, or the 'word' as the poetic function, and learning the ecstatic, sexual and shamanic magic of *seidr* from the goddess, Freyja: One wonders how. Odin also undertook a self-sacrifice on an ash tree where he pierced himself with a spear and in ecstatic trance retrieved the runes from the underworld. This limited overview of Odin shows the strong relationship he has to the British Woden and Myrddin, or Merlin, such that they seem regional variations of a central shamanic, mythic and prophetic archetype. It is in such company that Merlin should be considered.

The actual utterances in *Prophecies* remain obscure. Although they can be seen as metaphors for and predictions of events of the 12[th]C, they become quite cosmic with astrological symbolism and the use of classical mythic material. There is even the impression that they resemble a creation story and predict the end of the world, thus overlapping Biblical prophecy, which by foreshadowing the New Testament story carries a strange and parallel perspective of Merlin himself. This creation:destruction imagery is present in the first half of my Original Dream and is also present in the birth-death cycle of Merlin's life.

The Birth-Death Cycle of Merlin

Merlin's father is unknown, or so we are led to believe. This rather open-ended situation has, of course, led to him being identified by Christian hands as demonic, which then, unfortunately, becomes the standard default position. Accustomed as we are now to Christian gloss, I am going to put this interpretation to one side and ask what it might be obscuring. Because in Geoffrey's account he is simply absent, unknown.

Before resorting to Christianisation, Geoffrey's account draws on pre-literate Anglo-Celtic oral sources, with some reference and continuation of Nennius and the earlier Gildas (a contemporary of Arthur, if ever he existed, because Gildas does not mention him), both men of the cloth. Later in the 12thC, an Anglo-Saxon poet, called Layaman, rendered Geoffrey's account into Old English and also drew on similar non-Christian sources. What makes his poetic account of interest is that he identifies Merlin's father as an *elf* as I have independently done, prior to finding this out. This is quite a significant contrasting picture to the Christian demonic incubus, but may point to a truth. Incubi and succubi were considered to consort with humans; accounts of women being impregnated by incubi are legion, and many a man seems to have had an otherworldly succubus with whom he had intimate relationships: There seems to have been a lot of traffic between the worldly and otherworldly realities.

Yet this is the stuff of myth and legend worldwide. It is simply that here Layaman identifies such otherworldly beings as elves. This leads us into quite a different world to the one presented to us by Christianity. It is neither alien or demonic, it simply is an ever-present reality that interpenetrates ours, or vice versa. Specifically, such a notion of an absent father is a core element of many global myths of an exceptional or spiritually enlightened being; Jesus is but one example, his story resting as it does – like that of Merlin – on prophecy.

Certainly, the first part of my Original Dream is prophetic and relates to the immediate history of Hiroshima, but also to the broader creation mythology of many of the world's religions; the birth out of nothing or, in my case, the maternal womb of the Pacific Ocean. This progresses in the second part to the emergence of the father from the mists, having been previously unknown, although the mother and son were to me. Is this man an elf? Is that what the wounded Fisher King is? Am I to rejuvenate and rehabilitate him? I am starting to sound a bit like Perceval...

Up until and including Geoffrey, Merlin and his various alter egos simply exit the stage after the birth of Arthur; whose birth circumstances are not dissimilar to the above commentary and resonate with Merlin's own birth, to a large degree. For this reason, I am going to take the Arthurian story no further, although I will refer to intersecting features and circumstances like his birth, death, relationship with otherworldly women, and images like the Round Table when appropriate. In general, it is primarily a medieval creation and does not serve the purposes of this account, except where it may reflect certain features or endorse particular points. Effectively, the Arthurian legends and cycle is a story on its own that Merlin has been co-opted into, beyond the magical engineering of Arthur's birth.

Similarly, I am going to dismiss the accounts of Merlin's death as being due to the actions of a seductress keen to learn his art, using her sexuality to beguile and entrap him; curiously though, and like Arthur, he passes to an alternative *somewhere else*, but does not die in the physical sense. In the source material, there is no account of his death, except vague historical references (such as Lailoken), or as an elaboration of the mythic and symbolic *triple death* and its spiritual connotations. Incidentally, this was the case with Jesus, who was similarly interred, resurrected, and not seen to actually die. Intriguingly, Jesus was also surrounded by women more than by men during this episode.

In Geoffrey's later account of *Vita*, and in contrast to his unspecified literary exit in *Prophecies*, he does not die but exists in retreat with his companions. So where does this entrapment theme come from, given that we can now relatively dismiss the Christianised glossed version? Maybe his father, the elf, provides a hint. Also, there are the parallel myths and spiritual systems of other northern peoples to draw on, specifically Scandinavian and Teutonic.

In these systems women feature significantly. The goddess Freyja taught Odin *seidr* magic, which includes sexuality, as well as going some way to explaining Odin's gender ambiguity; somewhat strange for the principal god to be in the supposedly highly-masculinised Viking era. Even Uther in *Excalibur* when confronting Merlin, taunts him with his lack of knowledge of sexuality, culminating in telling him he would not know about desire, because "you are not a man!"

This sexual ambiguity is reinforced later in the movie, as Morgana entraps Merlin, saying, "you're not a god, you're not a man, I shall find a man and give birth to a god." Intentionally or otherwise, this could also be seen to refer to Merlin's parentage and that he is somehow *between* the states of godliness and manliness; although used in a derogatory manner here by Morgana, such an in-between state could refer to the marginality or liminality that ritual explores in spiritual pursuit, and maybe here referred to magical gifts. Of further interest is that Morgana's pregnancy will subsequently mimic Arthur's – the 'man' she finds – but it is hardly a god she gives birth to; the incest with its transgression of taboo are a palpable fault-line. Mordred's conception is from magic of a more self-serving kind directed toward power that ultimately fails; yet I wonder if this is but a darker and more obvious reflection of the *flaw* that brought down Camelot and ended the Age.

So, it may be that as part otherworldly being, Merlin simply disappears from the world and that the various female images may represent his own femininity, or other more objective personages who figure in it, maybe acting as portals. Alternatively, he may have had a female consort, a Julie, as a soror mystica. In this alchemical vein, and like Odin, his inner union of masculine and feminine may have rendered him genderless and "not a man". Or, as in Norse mythology, she could have been a Valkyrie who takes him from life back to the Otherworld; in this case, Valhalla, where resurrection is a given.

These are all various possibilities and maybe they all contain part of the truth, and point a finger toward what is ultimately a mystery.

INTERMISSION

If the reader has arrived at this point in this inquiry with the numerous questions that I have raised, often in a cyclic and sometimes repetitive manner – as well as those that this material would inevitably raise in any reader – he or she may wonder what has been achieved and where this narrative is going. This may be because I have had similar concerns at various points in the exposition, which is inevitable as I see it. This work is really a kind of journalistic narrative; an inquiry that has been and remains open-ended. I am letting it evolve as I write it and with it any insights and conclusions, it does not have an intentional goal or outcome. This is because my narrative is tracking something that is greater than myself. It is a process, and what it will ultimately reveal is not, as yet, entirely privileged for me to see; although because I have a prophetic sensibility, I am trusting what is to be revealed will emerge as I write (as, I suspect, some has already).

The above may sound a little like an excuse, a confession of sorts, which would be a fair enough assessment. What I am doing is trying to weave my own story into the account, with an intuitive trust that in so doing I will display my own prejudices and flaws, and not have them hidden in the narrative as some sort of authority. I see this too often as the case and it is understandable why, but I believe we are in a period of human evolution where such personal exposure is essential, because it is part of the ongoing story; we are part of the creative process with whatever is being created in some evolutionary and spiritual sense. Personal revelation is part of that equation in this era, I believe, as it has the capacity to rejuvenate many repetitive themes.

My understanding of the archetypal perspective is that it is perennial, inherently self-regulatory and powerfully directive. The archetypal complex of the prophetic visionary and healer is present in all cultures as a symbol of the spiritual urge for change, renewal, transformation and the like. I contend that we have adopted figures from other cultures, most specifically the Middle-Eastern figure of Jesus, for reasons that do not now reside in the inherent archetypal pattern of the mystical and magical visionary; instead, this religious figure has become used and commonly exploited for social, cultural and political purposes. That these purposes have often been brutal and contrary to the archetype of the shamanic healer indicates how far we have become disconnected collectively from this same archetype; a review of religious history is salutary in this regard.

What I am contending is that we need to look within our own culture, history and mythology for these patterns and people who have manifested them, rather than look for imports, mytho-historical or modern. What I am also highlighting is that doing this through many disciplines that currently examine this possibility can be circular and redundant; what we need to do is explore it through the lives and creative or other expressions of people who are sensitive to this kind of manifestation. What I am further doing is putting myself in that category. This is not superiority or arrogance; I see it as a responsibility too often shirked.

In some respects, in my own life I see that I am making a *great return* as Merlin does at the conclusion of *Vita*. Having been drawn away from a rural upbringing into the vocation of medicine, I found that of the various binaries – body:mind, science:art, material:spiritual – I was inclined to the latter and became progressively more so. In this process various career paths, including paradoxically one as a Jungian analyst, seemed to reach a conclusion and drop away, sometimes in a disruptive manner.

Of what remains, healing seems to stand out to me, maybe more than is portrayed in Geoffrey's account, although it is there in the shamanic and magical framework in which Merlin properly resides. Many of the other features of this archetypal complex resonate both within Merlin (and myself), such that he can be seen as a personal expression of it in Geoffrey's vision. This is one reason I found myself focusing on Geoffrey's rendering of Merlin, as it seemed to mark a juncture, a transition point. In the stories were some relevant accounts from history, such as Nennius, but there is also a considerable Celtic undercurrent from varied sources once the accretions that Geoffrey glossed in his account are teased out.

This is where the modern story of Merlin starts; it is familiar to us and, apart from reference where relevant, I will not follow it further. This is because I am more interested in tracking the archetypal features beyond history and re-establishing myth and fable as a fundamental. They operate within us anyway, it is just that with their relative denial and psychological reductionisms, they have given way to the structures of an often more personal nature with their attendant vested interests.

Not that I don't have mine, but I trust I am playing my hand fairly openly and providing a way to explore these interests in a similar manner to that with which I deal with others, if so inclined. Because, as I age, I see more how these deeper patterns drive and direct our lives; sometimes we align with them, most often – particularly in a rational, scientific and godless era – we do not. Much illness and disease I have experienced in my life and work is as a consequence of this failure, although in these states the seeds of transformation and redirection – getting *back on track* – are evident, particularly when one looks to undercurrents, such as dreams.

Which is what I have done here. I have and will continue to give dreams pride of place in this account with my personal input. They have revealed more depth and levels as I have written this narrative to date, which is one reason not to anticipate an outcome or conclusion, as yet. Hence, I can 'see' that Merlin's withdrawal from the world, and the ways this has been interpreted, will have a lot to inform me about this stage of my life in Part Two. I have used Geoffrey's accounts a little like I have my dreams, as a kind of background to and framework for this narrative. Both will continue to inform me as I progress, although Geoffrey's work will not be further added to. This is because he provides a clear picture of Merlin, or his various other personages, that consolidates on what has preceded it and with a British and Celtic flavour. His references to Arthur, in particular, are fleeting.

Within the century after Geoffrey, principally in the fifty years around the turn of the 13thC, there was an outpouring of work around Arthur and his legends that included Merlin, beyond the prior fleeting references. There was also his ongoing presence as the Arthurian legends progressed into the Grail Quest. Yet there is no direct reference to these to date in my dreams (mind you, there is little of Merlin either), except within the first half of the Original Dream. However, the image of the Grail portrayed here is unlike the accounts that flourished post-Geoffrey, with Wolfram of Eschenbach's notable exception, which will be examined in further detail in Part Two. Yet I have chosen Merlin as a deeper framework to my own life because he – or the archetype – resonates in so many ways; however, I accept the limitations of this choice and any criticism it may attract.

Instead, I will be providing a vision and version of the Grail that is unlike that in the popular imagination with its creative expressions. I find that this vision has much more to do with the mythic traditions of the Celtic and Northern peoples than the medieval one and its Christianisation. There has been some reference to this already, but more will follow and constellate around this version. I will be looking not only upon alchemy from this perspective, because although it historically is seen as medieval as a Tradition, it actually has a long prior and mystical history. As indicated, I will also be drawing upon the runes to support both this perspective and others.

Excalibur provides a Grail image that, on face value, is as we would expect; a chalice containing a revivifying fluid, wine, or maybe symbolic blood? But although supposedly staying true to Malory, the image is then grounded in a more Celtic vision. There is no Grail ritual or ceremony, ethereal women, or a wounded Fisher King (this figure becomes Arthur in the film); simply the connection of the Grail with Arthur's health – wounding (of a sexual nature), suffering, and ultimately healing – and the land in the sense of *Land*. This is the manner, by the way, that aboriginal people similarly refer to it in Australia, as *Country*.

Although not directly specified in the movie, I will be implying a deep and prior feminine association with the Land and femininity more generally, as well as issues of power and sexuality. Female images in *Excalibur* are generally restricted to Guinevere and Morgana, where other features are relatively condensed; for example, Morgana is generally a more nuanced and complex figure than the dark and manipulative lady of the movie, and neither the Lady of the Lake nor the women who convey Arthur, presumably to Avalon, are explored in any significant detail.

PART TWO

The Secret of The Grail

Introduction

The Holy Grail, henceforth simply the *Grail*, has intrigued me for decades. The adjective Holy is a Christian accretion, although somewhat paradoxically the word comes from the Old English *hal*, the language of the Anglo-Saxon period; intriguingly the words health, healing and wholeness derive from it.

Whilst Merlin has similarly captivated me more at a personal level, I had not been aware of any distinct association between these two themes. Many in my life have seen me as Merlin, possibly a consequence of my psychotherapeutic career and style of practice, as well as my regular underworld sojourns. Rather like Boorman and Pallenberg maybe, I began this narrative believing that it would be Merlin I would be exploring, but have found the Grail, along with Perceval and his namesakes, to have emerged in a demanding manner. Rather like the medieval Grail legends, I have sought – and am still seeking – the connection between Merlin and the Grail; a work in progress, it seems. I had anticipated this narrative to end here, yet I find myself feeling differently now and realise there is a further and deeper exploration of the Grail demanded, which I suspect will be through the eyes of Perceval.

As I came to the conclusion of Part One, I was clearly linking my life's story back to my dreams, yet found that my association of these with Merlin, as an archetypal figure, was becoming increasingly strained. Merlin was not as evident as I first considered, particularly as I lessened by gaze through his more exclusive archetypal lens and widened it. Maybe, as in the movie, he has done his job and it was time for him to depart; "there are other worlds," he tells Arthur in *Excalibur*. Instead, I could see the Grail and its more immediate legends around figures like the Fisher King coming more to the fore in my dreams.

The themes that connect these dreams are also embedded in the Grail legends, and to explore them in more depth I will need to appreciate Perceval further and enlist his help. Which leaves Merlin where? Has he simply been the ancestral évocateur that has kept me to task, and that now I have realised this, rather as he did with Arthur, has he now taken his leave? Time will tell; in *Excalibur* he did return after the Grail's attainment, and my prophetic gaze anticipates something similar here.

At various times I have tried to approach the Grail academically and creatively, but fallen away at what appeared to be a daunting task when so many before me had tried although not always successfully it seemed to me; this left a question mark for me that endured like a niggling splinter. The Grail field seemed well mined: What could I offer that could possibly be different? Watching *Excalibur* did not ease this discontent, as Merlin seemed to disappear with the advent of the Grail Quest, which was subsequent to Arthur's breaking of a sexual taboo in the conception of Mordred via his half-sister, Morgana, who had shape-shifted to the form of Guinevere to seduce him. This is a linking resonance to his own conception via Uther and Ygraine, indicating at least a cyclic nature to the unfolding events with a further transgression thrown in. Unlike Lancelot, there is no attempted healing of Arthur's subsequent wounded state, as he and the land languishes; did Merlin not know? It is these events that initiate the Grail Quest by the Knights of the Round Table to heal Arthur and with him, the Land, which appear to be the consequence of breaking the taboo… or is there more?

Merlin then appears later, after the Quest has been completed. He is now a distinctly Otherworldly figure who on Arthur's behalf, magically interferes to deal with his former captor, Mordred's mother Morgana, and help engineer the setting of the last battle before Arthur's physical and potentially terminal wounds have him escorted to Avalon. Merlin is a linking figure, but not directly so as he has no direct part in the Quest, rather it is to help guide Arthur further. These events in *Excalibur* are a product of the writers' imaginations and testify to the way they see the connection of Merlin with the Grail; peripheral, surrounding, but not direct when he would seem to have the appropriate capabilities to be able to effectively interfere.

Yet following Geoffrey, there was spawned a multitude of works about the Grail, with one of the first by Robert de Boron using Merlin as a linking figure with the now Christianised British history, as well as with Arthur and the Grail legends. There he remains for some, even to Malory's concluding work centuries later. I did not know what to make of this, or how to tackle it; my story as Merlin seemed complete with Part One. Then I recalled the *Sacrificial Dream* that I will come to, as well as seeing that my memoir and journalistic style might be the entry portal I needed. Because it always felt to me, as to others, that the significant stream of healing and death-rebirth cauldrons in Celtic and the Germanic Pagan traditions was superseded and glossed by Christian reworkings. They had seemingly languished beyond the written word, probably only available to those with a mythic and poetic sensibility. These features may, by now, be somewhat clearer to any religiously open-minded soul.

From the onset, I will partially reveal my hand... even to myself. Using dreams as a starting point, I will be taking the Grail story away from the seemingly common understanding that the vessel itself is the cup off the Biblical Last Supper, hence representative of the chalice used in the Eucharistic Mass. This impression has almost become established fact, and whilst it represents a Christian esoteric theme, it does not fit the core legend. The association of the cup with the lance that was used to pierce Jesus' side on the cross has more relevance, particularly with its blood association. Blood, as in lineage or bloodline, is another interpretation of the Grail, playing a bit on interpreting *San Grail* (Holy Grail) or *San Greal* with *Sang Real* (Royal blood). The spelling here is simplified and unified; there are alternatives that lead in many directions. The lance is of significance, yet to be discussed; although it is present at various points in the movie, including Mordred's euphemistic penetration of his father with it in *Excalibur*. The less tangible and least acknowledged possibility of the Grail, though maybe most accurate and pertinent to my inquiry given the Original Dream, is something *precious*; it thus provides an interesting word association with the ring in Tolkien's *The Lord of the Rings*.

In my understanding, Merlin's enduring presence does not point in the Christian and its Grail direction, rather it is toward pre-Christian and pre-historical sources. I will be looking at these to which I believe he more accurately refers us, although I am on common ground with others here. Whilst Christianity with its use of the Grail tries to point us forward in time, Merlin's continuing presence points to the past for what we have lost and need to retrieve, or maybe more accurately and esoterically, redeem and heal.

Although present in myth and other legends, usually of an oral nature, I will be relying on a healthy dose of intuition and the creative imagination in this venture. I could be putting the cart before the horse here and reaching conclusions about the Grail that may be premature and a reaction to the overall medieval and Christian position, rather than exploring the background and archetypal foundations that precede this. It may simply be better to start there and see what unfolds, so I would like to return to the first part of the Original Dream. Here's a recap:

I am looking at the sea from high above, as if on a map; it's the Pacific Ocean. A new island is emerging; it is called Hiroshima. It is a city island and I am now in the city square surrounded by old and gracious buildings. In the centre is a fountain. The sculpted centrepiece is like an organ-pipe cut at an angle at the top. As I gaze at it and look, almost seeing through it, it becomes a vast octagonal jewel.

At the time of the dream, I was just about to begin my Jungian analysis, so I saw it through this more psychological lens, as elucidated by my analyst. I really had little framework to see it any other way then, as dreams were a new area of exploration and for many years this Jungian orientation was the way I looked at and explained them. Any prior religious input for me was relatively passive and benign, and hadn't moved into anything intrapsychic. However, once I grasped this spiritual dimension beyond, yet also inclusive of the psychological, my view of dreaming and its significance changed and – I consider – matured accordingly. My prior knowledge of the Grail was basically drawn from the nursery, and alchemy I was yet to discover, which makes the dreaming process all the more interesting as such frameworks add appreciably to the understanding of them, as I trust will continue to be revealed. Seemingly, the dreaming process had pre-existing knowledge of this symbolism, which I find intriguing and challenging, as well as being in and of itself quite Jungian.

My analyst was a woman; a university lecturer in the arts; Christian; and what I would call a 'classic' Jungian. I mention these facts because it forms a background in which to context any insights I had at that time as I can recall them now, given the intervening lengthy period of time. Most of these insights and interpretations were not recalled from my therapeutic session, but a subsequent lecture given by her where this dream was discussed amongst those of others; although it was only the part immediately above that was presented, as I recall.

Jung posits a central archetype that he calls the *self* – a little confusingly to me given other psychological and commonplace views of this term – and sees it as the ordering principle that effectively unites the unconscious (both personal and collective) with consciousness; the ordering principle of the latter is the *ego*, incidentally. It is this '*self*' that effectively directs the *individuation process*, which he sees analysis to facilitate and support. Dreams and other products of this so-called unconscious are considered to be mediated and interpreted by the analysis, thus assisting the individuation process, rather than it being directed by the analyst. This archetypal *self* manifests in particular patterns and images, foremost amongst these are mandalas and principally these are in quadrated imagery. This *self* (as earlier stated, I will continue to italicise this Jungian concept to differentiate it from other similar definitions of the term) is seen as synonymous with *wholeness* in the individual, that is seen as more important than any idea of perfection, purity, and the like: It may be recalled the wholeness is etymologically related to both holy and healing.

The image of the quadrated city square, central fountain, and doubly-quadrated jewel could be considered a complex image of the *self*, to which I have provided personal and other associations in Part One. However, beyond these personal associations, it is what the symbols themselves reveal that provide a context and *amplify* the dream with material from more archetypal sources. In brief, I have seen these as feminine and Celtic, with birth and sexual imagery, and a central symbol that is a stone or jewel and is *precious*.

Now here is the leap, as I am going to anticipate what is to follow by saying that the Grail is effectively a *self*-image and not primarily existent in space-time; it is relatively consistent in its representation, manifesting in image, idea and affect, rather than material reality. To me, this Grail is a symbolic precious stone or vessel and accords more with the alchemical and Pagan themes that I favour. Interestingly, whilst most Grail accounts that followed Geoffrey flourished mainly from the French region of Europe, there is one work – *Parzival* by Wolfram von Eschenbach – that has similar imagery to mine for the Grail with the symbolic input of alchemy, as well as a religious perspective that is not limited to Christian Europe. Wagner was later to build on this theme in his operas.

I will return to all this, but in the meantime, I want to take the dream out of the exclusively Jungian context I was given and have briefly outlined here and connect it with broader and deeper features of my own psychic experience. I also want to continue to connect the psychological concept of the *self*, according to Jung, to the Grail; although there is more to be elucidated here when the other disciplines I have outlined are employed as well, even to different terminology. And I contend this is how Jung would have it; individuation is not simply a psychological process.

At this point in the narrative, various alternatives presented themselves. Having returned to the Original Dream to highlight its centrality and significance, I had once again opened up the whole area of the Grail for examination. Was I to pursue a chronological and academic inquiry, then the pathway would have been through writers such as Chrétien de Troyes and Robert de Boron into the Grail questing and adventures that are associated with the fictional Arthurian legends, hence occasionally linking in Merlin in a similarly medieval guise.

Now we are in distinctly medieval territory, where the politics of Kings and Courts, the Crusades and Christianity, absorbs this material to the point that it becomes disconnected from its pre-historical and Pagan past, except via the tenuous thread of Merlin's now fictionalised and potentially rehabilitated (i.e. Christianised) presence. Amongst others, the Cistercian Order's influence stands out and the association of the Grail with the celebration of the Eucharist through its supposed usage at the Last Supper becomes a given.

This Grail is often combined with its other featured presence to contain the blood from the Roman centurion-inflicted spear wound in Jesus' side at the Crucifixion, even though there is no mention of this event in the synoptic Gospels. However, the alternative pathway of the lance-inflicted wound is also present in the Grail symbolism and makes more sense to me; it also – minus the religious connotations – mirrors much in my further dream imagery. Though this avenue of the Grail history is less emphasised, it is obviously easy to associate the two events in the Passion, being the Last Supper and the Crucifixion, through the agency of the Grail as a chalice. And this has been done to the point that the view of the Grail being anything other than a holy Christian relic is anathema to most and simply incredulous to others.

So, here I would like to restore some balance and seemingly set the record straight by distinguishing the esoteric and mystical branch of Christianity from its exoteric religious cousin. The former, to my mind, connects us with the pre-Christian Pagan Traditions with common imagery; the latter is of the world, power, politics and institutional control. This latter branch I may refer to, but will generally eschew. In *Excalibur* the Grail's origins and nature beyond simply being a chalice are absent. This in itself is noteworthy, given the movie supposedly follows Malory.

The Passing of Merlin

Although commonly euphemistic for dying, I am not using *passing* selectively in that manner. Merlin may temporally, although arguably, have passed, but I contend that he is not necessarily *dead*, as in *passed away*. Merlin is an archetype; archetypes do not die. They may disappear into the psychological unconscious or Celtic Otherworld and exert their influence from there, when denied or out of favour in any particular time. And maybe that is what happened when the Grail emerged in response to demand into the Arthurian legends for healing the Land. In the movie, Merlin seems to be withdrawing from the 'affairs of men' when Arthur is King and becomes married, but he continues into the Grail legends in a different guise to the one outlined to date, exerting his influence in another manner. The reasons for this are speculative, as will be this whole section. But first I will start with what we have about Merlin and his *withdrawal* – a word I will now use to avoid ambiguity – in the written material already explored.

Merlin literally does ultimately withdraw in Geoffrey's *Vita* into some sort of retreat mode. His prophetic gifts are put aside and somehow given or returned to his sister, possibly being the feminine background from where they may have originated, as he retires with his companions in a strangely Jungian pattern of the *self*. I do not find this 'strangeness' invalid, it is just the rather awkward manner in which this happens with the introduction of previously unknown figures. I have seen these figures as aspects of Merlin and, once gathered together, they can integrate in a symbolic representation of unity and wholeness. Psychologically, this all makes sense. In this scenario, no physical death is described.

Instead in the shadows lurks Lailoken, with his triple death at the hands of a vengeful Queen. It is of interest that this is a consequence of a sexual misdemeanour on her part; well, from a conventional religious perspective, but maybe not to a Celtic sensibility. That the triple death may be symbolic and initiatory is relatively ignored, yet it litters history and the imagination, particularly as none of the components are definitively terminal in and of themselves; falling, suspension and immersion can all be seen in both a literal and symbolic light. In Geoffrey's *Vita* there is no literal death of Merlin.

Instead, we have a collection of various endings that seem coloured by the respective authors and the audience to whom they intend to appeal. Boorman and Pallenberg condense this in *Excalibur* to a power rather than a sexual seduction, which is juxtaposed with Arthur's confrontation of Guinevere caught in flagrante with Lancelot. There are some visionary images of this latter scene portrayed by Merlin to Morgana whilst within the dragon's domain. There is also one of a blond woman with a knight, who may be Morgana in her anticipated seduction of Arthur or even a reference back to her mother, Ygraine with Uther. In other words, the sexuality is around Merlin, but not directly involving him; the seduction with Morgana is based on power. These dynamics of sex and power are embedded in themes of transgression, revenge and magic.

The general theme of the medieval authors is that Merlin is erotically seduced by Morgana, or her various namesakes, to obtain his power. Also, that he is sexually or emotionally naïve and susceptible to such seduction. This a position that Boorman and Pallenberg relatively eschew; "You are not a man" were Uther's earlier words, implying he does not know such things and is not thus susceptible, so emphasising the power and magical dynamics. Although there is the extensive and often confused area of sexuality to yet explore, particularly with the varying and often contrasting Pagan and Christian perspectives, the implication – in the movie via the mechanism of the Charm – is that it is possession of magical power which is at stake here; sexuality itself is involved with power and procreative politics, rather than the erotic and love.

The condensed image is that Merlin is trapped when his magical power is taken from him. Although given literal representation – in a cave, underground, in a rock – this is metaphoric, as the bars to any release are psychic, not physical. In Boorman and Pallenberg's case, it is Arthur's love and his need that liberates Merlin. Love is a quiet feature that runs through *Excalibur* and may yet unite the differing Pagan and Christian positions. At this point, however, Merlin is ineffectual because of the wiles of the feminine; a strange inversion of the specifically Celtic and more broadly Pagan position… and even Geoffrey generally in *Vita*, in spite of the fact that this Merlin is supposedly married. More broadly then, this inversion bespeaks Christianity's exertion of power over, or taken from the Pagan, as well as its position with sexuality.

What is interesting is that, in spite of the Church's attempts in dealing with areas like the Pagan and the feminine, Merlin persists in some authors into the Grail accounts: It seems this esoteric and mystical branch of Christianity almost demands it, if not simply the various poetic and fictional authors feeling the need to retain a pre-Christian continuity. He has also, in the last couple of centuries, after a seeming hiatus, returned into the hands of poets and other creative avenues, too numerous to mention. In some sort of archetypal manner, he is still alive it seems.

Which means what? I return to my avowed archetypal perspective: The archetype of Merlin does not die, it passes into the modern 'unconscious', which is where Christianity would have him confined. It even uses a feminine agency to do this... how deceitful is this? But he is not dead. An archetype exists beyond space-time; is powerful and self-regulatory, and has a latent bipolarity. If denied or rejected, this polarity can be dark and potentially destructive, as in the forces unleashed in the wars of the 20thC, attributed by Jung to the metaphoric or literal shadow of Wotan (the Germanic Odin, or Woden).

In creative hands, Merlin is getting a more sympathetic hearing, as evidenced in the movie and the likes of TH White, Tolkien and many poets; he is being brought back to 'consciousness' and informing us still. Maybe it is prescient to say that our love has brought him back, or that the agencies of exoteric religion are losing their grip, or even that this is assisted by the return of the feminine (although I suspect all have their place): But back he is. Handle with care, *Excalibur's* Merlin would advise.

Which is what I have tried to do here, and a change has taken place. The examination of my own material to date has made me realise that while Merlin may be the archetypal figure who is directing my fate, it is more Perceval who appears to be fulfilling it in my actual life. I found myself somewhat constrained in trying to associate Merlin actually *in* the Original Dream, although I recognise his presence in somehow *directing* it (maybe a little like Boorman). So, the figure in the garden – that memory of yore – is not personal in the same way the psychoanalytic memory was and is; it is more transpersonal. With this subtle but deep shift of emphasis, I wonder how I will experience Merlin's relationship with Perceval and the Grail legends as I move forward?

There is a relative discontinuity between Parts One and Two, which is not directly of my making. It centres around the figures of Merlin and Perceval. Merlin, in the historical accounts, has clear connections between the Celtic and medieval worlds, even if the medium has now changed from verbal to written as the primary manner in which this expressed. When we come to the end of the 12thC and the manifestation of the Grail corpus, there appears to be more concern for matters of the temporal *present*. This is clearly evident in the Grail legends, where contemporary issues around issues like spirituality, love and morality are being explored, and sometimes contrasted with the heathen and amoral perception of the pre-Christian past that Merlin – particularly in his *passing* – exemplifies. In contrast, and although there is a connection to the Welsh Peredur, Perceval and other Grail legend figures now make up the medieval world.

Yet there is something more subtle going on here, to my mind. I have expressed elsewhere how I do not see space and time as part of the same continuum: Space I see as having substance in the material world (earth, if you like), whereas time is more fluid (watery). Other analogies could be space:time is equivalent not only to earth:water and hence structure:process, but even self:soul (the daily consciousness and psychological self, and not the Jungian archetypal *self*). I hold this to be the case, that time is a quality of the soul and should be seen in that light, not reduced to concrete rationality.

In this way, Perceval can be seen to be moving *forward* in time; an evolving figure and expressive of the concerns of the spirit as they unravel in areas like religion and ethics. By way of contrast, Merlin seems to move or direct our view of him *backward* in time. This is something that a modern writer on Merlin, TH White, has explored and – dare I say it – this principle crops up in Dr Who. Merlin is connecting us with the *past*, but in an archetypal and paradoxical manner, directing us toward the *future*. I wonder if such a Merlin could be considered a genuine time-traveller?

In my opinion, there is a marked change in awareness at this time in the medieval era; it was a transitional, the old was going through a metaphoric death and something new was emerging…

maybe under Merlin's tutelage. Up until this period, the prime method of storytelling was auditory and collective. Imagine the scenes of a Bard recounting stories around a fire to an illiterate group, adding his own inflections in a theatrical way. This is obscure to us now, as we only have the redacted versions that were committed to writing, with a potential second level of obfuscation. I mention this, because I experience such written second-hand accounts of oral narratives often to be bland, with the bare minimum of reporting and no embellishment; they feel dry and emotionless, which doesn't help discern some of the conveyed facts. Maybe the passion is when they are read to an audience, demanding the orator's skill?

With writing, beyond the preferences of the author, his (not usually a *her* in that time) sources and the circumstances of the time, there is the inclusion now of *feeling* in *visionary* form – hence available to the private individual – that adds to the nuance and subtlety of the tale, which was only previously available in the *auditory* form and not in the written accounts, unless enacted as well. Once writing escaped the strictures of Latin, this expression would only have increased. I mention all this because it is important to include the *internal emotional* dimension in this transitional phase, rather than it being projected onto the 'stage', so to speak. In my opinion, there is no real change in consciousness without emotion's inclusion at the individual level, amplified with collective relevance. Symbolically, at least, maybe it is significant that Geoffrey and hence Merlin, brought these changes to the British Isles and then retired.

I am relatively dismissing the more specific accretions around power and sexuality (and hence the feminine) in Merlin's withdrawal, although they will need to be given a broader more psychologically balanced and Pagan spiritual airing. How is his withdrawal to be viewed then? There is a pattern that weaves its way through these various viewpoints, and that is that Merlin withdraws somehow into the Land and/or the *beyond*. *Excalibur* gives this similar impression, with it being more the Underworld, if the imagery is considered. Merlin specifically equates this with the coils of the *dragon* and hence the invocation of the Charm, which is uttered here in a transfer of power scenario of the movie's making. Consideration should also be given to Merlin's parentage from the earlier prophetic youth character in *Prophecies*. Again, the Christian accretion of the devil or an incubus can be stripped away and his father pictured more as an *elf*, as in the poet Layaman, when a more Celtic or Anglo-Saxon perspective is taken at this period in time.

If all these apparent hints and suggested scenarios are placed together, it seems more like Merlin is making a return of sorts; a completion of a cycle. There are resonances of this in others, most specifically Arthur, both in the unusual nature of his conception and his own passing, except this is across water rather than in the earth. However, both are natural feminine elements, and the destination of *Avalon* may have some commonality. I propose that Merlin is returning to the Otherworld, the world of Faery, and the backward movement to a time past but archetypally ever-present that I have explored above. In this venture, the feminine would be supporting and helping him, rather like Arthur, as assistance is required in his case. Even the Christian scenario indicates only entrapment; its mechanisms in this process are more an inditement of magic (and sex), but not actual death in the physical sense.

There remains an interesting paradox in Merlin's withdrawal. With Geoffrey, there is no death in the literal sense, so he does not provide a template for the various ensuing and varying accounts. Also, Geoffrey seems to rehabilitate Myrddin from his association with Lailoken, hence with the latter's apparent death. Why should he do this? And why have the romance writers who subsequently started to document the Arthurian and Grail legends not chosen to metaphorically bury Merlin and his alter egos this way? It would seem to have been convenient and a clear demarcation between the pre-Christian and Christian eras. Why take him into the Grail's world at all and necessitate finding a different way of getting rid of him?

There are various ways to look at this. One of the more obvious is that the various writers, rather like Geoffrey, had a pre-Christian sensibility and wanted to provide a connection with it. A second is Merlin moving beyond this sensibility, by becoming the victim of sexual and feminine forces that the Church wished to suppress; maybe his passing was sacrificial? If so, there is something of an irony here, linking him to Jesus and the Christ archetype. It is almost as if Merlin *cannot* be killed, even by the Church – he is an archetype, after all – and that he, or *we* find a way out of that entrapment, which may now be happening in our present time. In a psychological sense, there is the *return of the repressed* occurring or, in a more specific Jungian sense, the archetype has been talking to the visionaries and poets from his entrapped position and is now re-emerging to inform our time and its future direction.

Yet there is something else, and maybe it is within my dream and elements in *Excalibur* I have yet to arrive at, which is why the triple death of Lailoken was not used as a way of 'getting rid of him'? I suspect that there is something even more powerful in this possibility, in that it would associate Merlin too much with the Christian position of the Crucifixion, maybe as the central archetype of the Jungian *self* that Christianity has tried to pin entirely on Jesus (excuse the pun). The Church would then become relative and allow for the Pagan continuity that might arise, which it psychologically inevitably will when such repressive forces are used. Merlin, or even Woden as an alternative, as *the* Christ may just have been too much. Yet, somewhat ironically and paradoxically, in trying to rid us of these alternatives and thus making Jesus the one-and-only, and rather like with Pilate and the Jewish authorities, it is Merlin's resurrection that is instead promoted.

Incomplete though this inquiry might be, it is not finished, and the triple death may be a significant symbolic focus in what is yet to emerge.

Initial Representation of the Grail

Within Excalibur

There are many difficulties using *Excalibur* as the source material for the Grail legend. Although claimed to be from Malory's 15thC *Le Morte d'Arthur*, this Grail sequence seems to be more a continuation of the prior story up to this point in the movie, which is now around two-thirds of the way through. It would take me too far afield to try and reason fully the anomalies and inconsistencies, which I will not try and do; instead, I will simply see it as Boorman and Pallenberg's interpretation and put it in some context.

I am using *Excalibur* to have a foundation in understanding of the Grail at the close of the medieval period, because – to my mind – it has distinct connections back to the beginning of this period when the legends were first penned, then even to times prior. For example, in Malory's work, and following the Christian-based legends, it is Galahad and not Perceval who in the movie attains the Grail. Also in Malory, his name is spelled *Percival*. This effectively takes the portrayal in the movie back to the original written source of Chrétien de Troyes in the 12thC, which is where I will return to when I move forward with the significance of the Grail in my account. I find this confluence of time periods significant on the part of the screenplay writers.

Of these many anomalies and inconsistencies in the movie, some can be put down to the limitations of the art, the preference of the writers, and their seeming desire to have Merlin as the main feature. And even if the latter is not directly the case, Williamson's acting portrayal of Merlin steals the show. This would appear to diminish the Grail segment, although the imagery and story, as given in the movie, do highlight some intriguing features that I find relatively enchanting (word carefully chosen). It also – intentionally or otherwise – manages to de-gloss Malory's Christianisation and present a simple theme of the transition from Paganism to Christianity without unnecessarily eulogising the Grail legends in a Christian manner.

Instead, the Grail is associated with Arthur, even down to the shape-shifting of the Grail image to that of him as the Grail King, when Perceval answers the question. The Grail is seen as the agent that will restore the King's connection to the Land and its health and vitality; this is an ancient theme indeed. This is also the basis of the Grail questions and Perceval's answers, an interesting inversion of the various legends where it is Perceval's responsibility to ask questions of the Grail King. There is no ritual or procession, feast, Fisher King or Grail maidens; the wounded King is Arthur himself, with his wounding in the Church subsequent to his magical seduction by Morgana and Mordred's birth with the ensuing disconnection of the King and Land. The wounding is dragonesque, being lightening, and the location in his body is not defined, although with this pattern it is not difficult to see it as genital; although in a more symbolic light, it could be the heart. The lightening also resembles or could symbolise a lance or spear. Such relative obfuscation around sexuality is an interesting feature in a movie otherwise relatively frank in visual imagery, particularly the brutality of war and attendant violence.

All this as may be, it is Perceval's journey I want to highlight. Perceval is introduced to the audience through an encounter with Lancelot on one of the latter's solo adventures away from court (and hence avoiding Guinevere). Perceval presents as naïve and young, though he pleases Lancelot sufficiently to be allowed to accompany him back to court at Camelot. After a period of menial duties, he brazenly attempts to defend Guinevere's honour prior to Lancelot's appropriate intervention, although he has also inadvertently become knighted by Arthur in this process. He then takes his place at the Round Table. With Arthur's wounding and demand that the knights seek the Grail for his and the Land's healing "to the edge of... within", he sets off. This remark itself rings my psychospiritual alarm bells, in that either Boorman or Pallenberg, or both, are looking at the Grail Quest in a relatively psychological or spiritual and not primarily religious manner.

Eventually, and after many years, Perceval finds himself in Morgana's presence. But in failing to be dissuaded from the Quest and with Mordred's demand, he is hung by the neck from a tree in addition to other prior knights, already expired. An act of apparent fate, seemingly like his attaining of knighthood, brings about the breaking of his noose and he falls to the ground. However, whilst near death he has had a vision of the Grail and is asked disembodied questions about the secret of the Grail and whom it serves. He runs from this visionary confrontation in silence and apparent fear, as he simultaneously falls from the tree. This leaves the impression that he has had a near death experience and a vision in an altered state of consciousness. He bemoans his apparent lapse and continues the Quest.

After an encounter with a dying knight, murdered by a now grown Mordred, he is encouraged to continue the Quest. He then encounters a wild-looking, dishevelled and presumably mad Lancelot amongst pestilent death, within a mourning and bereft community. The inference is that Lancelot's grief has brought him here, reinforced by having a goblet in his hand that may be alcohol, or a resonance with the Grail. Those with Lancelot, though under his direction, pursue, beat and push Perceval into a fast-running rocky stream where he is swept under and removes his armour. He arrives at the Grail castle as before, but unlike his first visit there, this time he is (relatively) naked and answers the questions associating the secret with Arthur and the Land, as a visionary Arthur assumes the Grail King's image. He then returns with the Grail and revives the physical Arthur with the drinking of its unspecified red contents.

The story now returns to Arthur in his final battle and killing of Mordred, his son, before he is conveyed away in the boat to – presumably – Avalon. The sword is simultaneously returned to the lady of the lake by Perceval.

Some comment has already been made about the screenplay and its connection to other sources; at least to Chrétien as the first known formal Grail Quest writer, but also other pre-Christian sources, including the Welsh stories of Peredur. Here I would like to look at how the movie portrays him, because I find it significantly initiatory, which is reasonably captured in the above brief outline.

There is a significant prior history to Perceval's encounter with Lancelot, not present in the movie and to which I will come, although his presentation as a bit of a fool – again recalling the relevant Tarot card – is an appropriate representation. His initiation into Lancelot's affection begins when he serves him a meal and is then allowed to accompany him to Camelot. His knighting – a seeming accident – is another initiatory step, where deeper forces surrounding his destiny and forthcoming spiritual role also play a part. Unfortunately, in his pursuit of the Grail, there is no female imagery or sexual reference – Morgana notwithstanding – which is a strong feature of the legends.

Perceval's major initiations are reserved for his Grail experiences. This is true to and consistent with the medieval legends, although in Boorman's hands the sequences immediately prior to each Grail encounter are quite revealing. Here, as elsewhere, I am impressed by the psychological depth of the screenplay, although I may beg to differ from it on occasion. What is remarkable to me is that the imagery repeats the triple death in a slightly altered form, possibly because there are just two steps of it in the Grail achievement in which the death is condensed.

The psychological is taken to the parapsychological in the first encounter. As already described: Hung by his neck from a tree, Perceval undergoes a near death experience that contains a vision of the Grail. Of interest, is that it is fear that thwarts his ability to answer the question, whereas in the legends it is his prior conditioning about silence in such circumstances with the consequence that he falls asleep. Why he should be fearful is unclear, unless he is in awe of the encounter... although this doesn't quite ring true to me. Yet the paranormality is true to accounts of such states and this, when allied with the sleeping themes in the legends, raises questions about states of consciousness. It also reinforces the earlier command of Arthur's to seek to the edge of *within*. Yet the overarching image of the suspension from the tree is what stands out, with his seemingly fortuitous release from impending death, it resonates with the second segment of the triple death.

The first and third triple death sequences are reserved for his second Grail encounter. On this occasion the background is disease, madness and death... and Lancelot maybe mirroring Arthur as his psychological shadow with his frenzied grief, in contrast to Arthur's extreme apathy and wasting that mirrors the Waste Land. The presence of the pseudo-Grail in Lancelot's hands, which he casts at Perceval in the river, is a nice touch. The rustic men who attack Perceval and push him with sticks and pitchforks into the river becomes the falling image of the triple death and a strange resonance of the Lailoken story, about which

I see no other reference in *Excalibur*. Then Perceval is cast down the river over rocks into a depth from whence he takes off his armour; a further initiation, accompanied by Wagner's music. Although I suspect that the writers are trying to catch a death-rebirth pattern here, it also resonates with the drowning of the triple death.

Now I find myself back at the questions I had – and have – surrounding Merlin's entrapment. The deep question I now have is that if Merlin's death – as Lailoken – were to be continued into the Grail legends, then does this resonate too much with the Crucifixion… is there something here the Church feared and maybe still fears, as indirectly enunciated a little earlier? Although Perceval's connection with the triple death is of Boorman and Pallenberg's creation, is there a Jungian synchronicity here? And, if so, what is the newfound resonance between Perceval and Merlin? Are these some of the questions that need to continue into the Grail legends, but were effectively headed off at the pass by the Church's influence?

As *Excalibur* appears to do as an undercurrent, it is here that I part ways with the more culturally and politically Roman – via the Church – direction of these narratives. I favour a more Germanic route and have Wolfram's *Parzival* to come to for this. This is not the only reason to get back to this 12ᵗʰC apparent bifurcation, something I believe others like Tolkien have done, but I do feel we have lost much in our over-identification with Christian, Roman, European and even Middle-Eastern influences at the expense of other aspects of our heritage, both historical and spiritual. I suspect that is why Merlin still lives and we do have to contend with Woden in this scenario, as an extension of Merlin backward in time and downward in depth.

Summary

The image of the Grail we are left with after *Excalibur* remains clearly a chalice containing a red fluid, like wine or blood. In spite of the other indications and impressions outlined above, this leaves the image as clearly the Christian one of the chalice; being either the cup containing Jesus' blood from the lance-inflicted wound on the cross, or the cup of the Last Supper... or both. In the background is a vague bloodline theme with Arthur's heritage and that it is an agent of *healing*, which in and of itself is *precious*.

This leaves me a long way from being decided what the Grail is and may look like; questions that strangely reflect those asked of the Grail seeker. Rather like some of the medieval works, I am now going to end this initial inquiry rather abruptly, as I believe we need to ask further about the Grail's seeker in the Quest. For this, I am going to move sideways from the movie to the first written account of the Grail written some fifty years after Geoffrey, in the late 12th century. The transition is quite smooth from one Perceval to another, making me believe this may have been the screenplay writers' inspiration in *Excalibur*.

Yet here is a salutary 20[th]C reminder by the poetic author of *The Waste Land*, TS Eliot, of a famous quote from his later *Four Quartets*:

> "We shall not cease from exploration
> And the end of all our exploring
> Will be to arrive where we started
> And know the place for the first time."

Grail Questers

Perceval

Perceval, the Story of the Grail is a romance by Chrétien de Troyes, unfinished, and written in Old French toward the end of the 12thC. Because it is seminal, I will be presenting Perceval in some detail that will reverberate through the following questers' stories and hence render them more briefly.

The following is a synopsis available online, with some minor editing on my part for clarity. Although relatively lengthy, it captures some of the themes and subtlety more abbreviated versions omit, I had initially thought I would need to write my own, until I came across this whilst researching another poem:

> *Perceval grows up in the Waste Forest in NW Wales, raised alone and in ignorance of knighthood by his mother. Five knights arrive and he marvels at their appearance, thinking they are God. They describe their knightly furnishings. One has been recently knighted by King Arthur, who is staying in Carlisle, in Cumbria NW England.*
>
> *His unnamed mother is distraught to learn he has met the knights, and tells him of his father, the knight Gahmuret, how he was wounded, lost his wealth, was come home. Perceval's two brothers became knights and died in combat, and Gahmuret died of grief. But*

Perceval can only think of becoming a knight, and leaves his mother with her reluctant blessing. She advises him to assist any lady in need, to serve ladies and maidens.

In an encounter with an unnamed damsel in a vermilion and striped tent, Perceval forces kisses from her and forcibly takes her ring, misinterpreting his mother's advice. The woman's lover returns, and accuses her of infidelity, resolving to punish her by making her go naked and on foot. He is also heading toward King Arthur's. King Arthur has fought and defeated King Ryon. He is at Carlisle, a castle above the sea.

Perceval encounters the knight in red armour who has laid claim to Arthur's land, and sends Perceval to bear a message to Arthur.

Perceval comes into Arthur's court, refuses to dismount, hurriedly asks to be knighted (but does not seem to wait for this to be done), and asks to be granted the armour of the Red Knight. The handsome but evil-tongued seneschal Kay mocks him, challenging him to get the Red Knight's armour, and Arthur rebukes Kay. A maiden (the queen's handmaiden, unnamed) laughs for the first time in six years, and Kay strikes her and also the court jester, who has prophesied "This maiden will not laugh until she has seen the man who will be the supreme lord among all knights."

Perceval returns to the Red Knight, demands him armour, and quickly kills him with a javelin through the eye. He is advised by Yonet and takes the knight's armour and horse – Yonet receives Perceval's own *horse. He sends Yonet with Arthur's stolen cup and a message to Arthur. The jester prophecies that Perceval will avenge the kick Kay gave him.*

Perceval rides away and comes to a castle by a river and the sea. He encounters a gentleman in ermine, Gornemant of Gohort, and they converse. Perceval asks for lodging, and Gornemant begins to teach him how to conduct himself as a knight. Perceval expresses concern about his mother, whom he saw faint as he was leaving her. The next morning, Gornemant gives him clothing and a sword, conferring on him knighthood. Gornemant advises Perceval to not be too talkative or prone to gossip, to find a maiden or woman whom he can console, and to go to church, and not to claim publicly that he was taught by his mother. Perceval departs to find his mother.

He encounters another castle, Biaurepaire, by the sea. There he finds a charming maiden Blancheflor whose followers are weakened by hunger and famine. She is Gornemant's niece. At night she comes innocently into the sleeping Perceval's bedroom and gets into bed with him, embracing him. She relates there will be an imminent attack by Anguingueron, the seneschal of the evil knight Clamadeu of the Isles, and that they have previously attacked and carried away many of her men. She will kill herself before allowing herself to be taken to Clamadeu. Perceval promises to help Blancheflor and asks only for her love in return. She stays the night with him in bed. The next morning, Perceval does battle with Anguingueron, whom he fells but spares after Anguingueron begs for mercy. Perceval orders him back to Arthur's court to serve the maiden that Kay struck.

Clamadeu learns his seneschal has been defeated. Perceval does battle with 20 of Clamadeu's knights and wins the day. Clamadeu's adviser suggests he wait it out and let the starvation inside have its effect. But a ship with wheat and provisions arrives. At last Clamadeu does battle with Perceval and is forced to beg for mercy. He also is sent back to Arthur's court to the maiden whom Kay struck. Clamadeu also releases all his prisoners. The two defeated knights appear before Arthur and his queen are staying now at Disnadaron in Wales. The two knights tell of their defeat by Perceval, and the jester again rejoices that he will be avenged. Arthur expresses regret that Kay drove Perceval away. The knights Girflet and Yvain hospitably escort the two new arrivals away.

Perceval departs Blancheflor, determined to find his mother. He encounters monks and nuns from the town, and speaks of his mother to them.

At a river, he sees two men in an anchored boat fishing, one of whom is the Fisher King. Perceval is unable to cross, and the Fisher King offers him lodging for the night. Perceval climbs up a cleft in the rock to the top of a hill where he arrives at a splendid castle with tower and hall. Inside, he sees a nobleman with greying hair seated on a bed, the lord of the castle (the Fisher King) who is unable to rise to greet him. A squire enters carrying a sword with engraved blade, and announces that the lord's niece has sent it to him – the lord gives the sword to Perceval. Another squire enters carrying a white lance on whose tip blood oozed and flowed down onto the squire's hand. Perceval refrains from asking about this lance, recalling Gornemant's admonishment. More squires bring in candelabras. A maiden brings in a grail held in both hands (for Chrétien, it is a serving dish), and the room becomes brightly illuminated (presumably because of the contents of the grail). Another brings in a silver carving platter. The grail is made of gold and set with precious stones – it and the platter are carried to another chamber. Perceval fails to ask who is being served by the grail. They dine at an ivory table. The grail returns borne in the opposite direction. Later that night, the Fisher King excuses himself and has to be carried off to his bedroom, and Perceval again fails to ask what ails him. The next morning, Perceval discovers that the hall is deserted and everyone has left. As he rides over the drawbridge, the drawbridge mysteriously raises up on its own.

He encounters a maiden beneath an oak tree. She holds a dead knight, whose head has been cut off by another knight that morning. She marvels that he stayed with the Fisher King. She says the Fisher King was wounded in a battle by a javelin through both thighs and is still in much pain, and that he seeks diversion from his pain by fishing. She rebukes him for not asking why the lance bled or what is done with the grail or who was being served by the grail and silver platter, saying he would have brought great succour to the king if he had. Perceval says as a guess that his name is Perceval the Welshman, but she renames him Perceval the wretched. She says much suffering will now befall him instead of what could have happened. She says she is Perceval's first cousin, was raised with him for many years, and that his mother is dead. Perceval offers to pursue her lover's killer. She warns him that the sword he was given could shatter in his moment of need, and that Trabuchet alone could fix it.

Perceval departs and soon encounters a weary palfrey [woman's horse] ridden by a wretched girl with torn clothing and lacerations. She recognizes Perceval as the man who stole the ring and kisses from her, and warns him that the Haughty Knight of the Heath will kill him just as he has earlier that day killed another knight. The Haughty Knight of the Heath arrives and tells his tale of how he suspects the Welshman lay with her. Perceval confesses he was the man, is challenged to a fight, and defeats the knight. He informs him of her faithfulness to him, and demands they both go to Arthur's court and the damsel that Kay struck. The couple rides on and comes before Arthur at Caerleon (SE Wales). Arthur frees him from his imprisonment and turns him over to his nephew Gawain. Arthur does not know Perceval's name, and resolves to set off from Caerleon in search of Perceval. Later, Perceval is near Arthur's camp, and is lost in thought on seeing three drops of wounded goose blood on the snow, which reminds him of his beloved Blancheflor. Sagremor informs Arthur that they have found a knight asleep on his horse. Sagremor challenges Perceval, and is defeated. Kay also challenges him, and breaks his collar bone and arm, just as the jester had foretold. The king takes pity on Kay and has the physician attend him. Gawain offers to go to watch how Perceval behaves and to bring him back through more diplomatic means. He approaches Perceval, and Perceval learns from him that it was the seneschal Kay whom he defeated and on whom he had wanted to have his vengeance. They become friends, and Perceval

*introduces himself as Perceval the Welshman. Gawain
says Perceval has fulfilled the prophecies of the jester
and the maiden. Perceval comes before the court, and
addresses the maiden, saying he will always come to her
aid. They return to Caerleon.*

*They encounter a damsel on a tawny mule and having
a beard and humpback. She taunts Perceval for not
asking the needed questions at the Fisher King's hall.
She is on her way to the Proud Castle. Gawain resolves
to help the maiden besieged on the peak of Montesclere.
Perceval however resolves to not rest until he has
learned who was served by the grail and why the lance
bled.*

[After a long tale of Gawain's pursuits, the Perceval tale resumes]:

*Perceval has gone five years without entering a church,
and has sent sixty defeated knights to Arthur's court. He
encounters knights and ladies on the trail, penitential.
They criticize him for bearing arms on Good Friday.
One pilgrim blames the Jews for the death of Christ.
They have gone to see a holy hermit, and Perceval wants
to do the same. With their directions, he arrives at the
hermitage, tells the hermit of his years of wandering,
and the encounter with the grail and the lance. The
hermit, Perceval's uncle, tells him how his mother had
died from sorrow at his departure, a sin which requires
repentance and which caused him to fail to ask about
the grail. The man who is served from the grail is the
hermit's brother, brother also to Perceval's mother, and
he believes the Fisher King is the man's son. He says the
grail is holy and sustains the holy man because it carries
a single consecrated host he has lived on this host for
twelve years. Perceval agrees to undergo penance and*

189

take a limited diet with the hermit, acknowledging
Christ and taking communion.

[Gawain tale resumes, after which the story abruptly ends.]
(Synopsis by Michael McGoodwin, online source.)

It is also left unfinished and in mid-sentence, leading scholars to believe that Chrétien either experienced a tragedy or died suddenly at this point; I am not so sure. Rather like Perceval, I have come on this story relatively innocently and a little surprised. Apart from the poem and various summaries of it, I have decided to deliberately retain my naïveté and explore it without recourse to anything written by other commentators. I will leave that until later, if it becomes necessary.

My first observations are that, without the Grail procession, I would be very surprised if the poem would have attracted the attention it did. The story is otherwise familiar in the context of the time, but the procession is a new introduction providing a haunting and enigmatic focus, so with its lack of completion it is easy to see why there was such an interest in concluding it. In so doing maybe the spiritual focus was continued, although progressively along more Christian lines (here and elsewhere I see Christianity as relatively synonymous with the Roman Church for the purposes of this account), with the connections to the prior and maybe still coexistent Pagan Tradition becoming progressively minimised.

I also wonder about the last paragraph of Perceval's meeting with the hermit; it feels Christianised to the point that I wonder if it is also added and even written by another hand, coming as it does book-ended by the adventures of Gawain. The *host* features strongly here, yet is not mentioned before; in fact, the prior account to this point is mystical, symbolic and ritualised, but not distinctly Christian like this final paragraph. I suspect there are arguments to the contrary expressed in academia, but the very fact it is questionably Chrétien's hand is itself significant to me. If so, maybe this might add to the mystery of the poem's lack of completion. Just thinking.

As a note: Gawain features frequently here and in other similar poetic renderings; he seems to be a psychological shadow figure to Perceval, a kind of idealised Knight. He may also be a precursor to the later Galahad as Grail achiever. I will generally be omitting his adventures hereon; they are relevant to the overall Grail corpus, but complicate my intention. The Grail has not been referred to as holy until then, and now both describes the hermit, and also the wounded King. The host is not mentioned until then and one gets the impression of the prior fare being food and drink in a more Celtic manner, as well as it referencing something more traditional.

Shortly after Chrétien wrote *Perceval* (he died in 1191) another French author, Robert de Boron, wrote *Joseph of Arimathea* and, somewhat intriguingly, *Merlin*. According to scholarship, works known as *Perceval* and *Morte Aru* were to complete his body of work. Robert is significant in that he links the Grail legend back to Jesus' time with *Joseph* and effectively commences the theme of the Grail being the cup of the Passion or Crucifixion story with which we are now collectively familiar. Effectively, this now bypasses the first millennium input from non-Christian sources.

Even as de Boron builds on Celtic material, in this process there are inevitably some resonances that remain, such as with Bron, Joseph's brother-in-law, who becomes the Grail's caretaker. He heads West to Britain with his entourage and his grandson, Perceval, becomes the Grail King. Now, by a play of words, Bron may be Boron himself. Alternatively, and even anyway, he could refer to Brân the Blessed and hence the head on the platter of Peredur's tale of the Grail, to which I will come. A further point is that in Chrétien's poem, "King Arthur has fought and defeated King Ryon"; is this Bron or even Brân, because Arthur does assume his place in London, in legend.

In many respects Robert's supposed history is a Chrétien continuation along a distinctly Christian path, with the introduction of the fabled Joseph and potential bloodline story, as well as how the Grail arrived in Glastonbury. Ironically, Robert refers to his work as a history, whereas the other Grail writers preferred to call their works a story, or are referred to as *romances*. Maybe it resonates because it is a template for the many modern variations of the Grail theme that abound in literature and film as pseudo-histories – and hoaxes. Perceval becomes a Christian apologetic in the various ongoing accounts after Robert, and Merlin is now considered a product of the devil's tryst with or rape of a virgin, and destined to become a redeemed Antichrist in the poems and future stories; a strange variation on healing, methinks. It is also a further argument for his ongoing presence… and demonisation.

There are various – at least four – continuations of Chrétien's story, as other poets and authors appear to scramble to complete the poem. Perceval morphs into Galahad and a progressively continental Christian tone becomes evident. Too numerous to mention, and not directly relevant to my account to further elucidate, are the works that comprise the *Vulgate Cycle* (alternatively known as the *Lancelot-Grail*) which has some prior reference to Merlin and Perceval, though in a Christianised context and under significant Cistercian influence. As these go along a more idiosyncratic path according to authorship and preferences, I will not be pursuing these further, although they form a major component of the vast *Arthurian Corpus* and are the subject matter of much of Malory's *Le Morte d'Arthur* and the (relative) close of an era, in a literary sense.

One exception to this rather generalised understanding is a strange work known as *The Elucidation of the Grail* written in the early 13thC, supposedly as a prologue to Chrétien's poem, although it significantly departs from it into areas of the feminine and Celtic world with a strong initiatory and redemptive theme; these elements will be returned to in my account, although not from this source. There are also accounts of vengeance and blood references, along with those of a more Otherworldly and dreamlike state of consciousness. Although not explored in detail, it seems to me to put Chrétien into a different context and direction compared to how the *continuation* authors and then others have taken the subject matter; maybe that was the *Elucidation* author's intent, because there are distinct similarities to what I am trying to achieve here.

There are a couple of more obscure themes that I am detecting when surveying the whole field of contribution in the brief period – around fifty years – of the works described. The first is the tension between the Roman and Germanic worlds, with the French being in the former Church camp in the Holy Roman Empire days from Charlemagne on, and the Germanic world with its Pagan Traditions. Effectively this is a continuation of a dichotomy that can be seen in Merlin's time of the 5-6thC and also highlighted in the later time period of the film *Excalibur*; to my mind, it continues still and this present work is testament to this as well as its potential reconciliation, or a healing process.

The second is the time period of the 8-9thC that attracted my attention with Nennius and Merlin in Part One. Charlemagne was crowned Emperor in 800 CE and was a powerful empire in Europe until the 12thC when, coincidentally, these poems started to appear. Rather like the Roman Church's success after the departure of the Roman Empire in Britain, I wonder how much the change in this religious balance in the 12thC is reflected in the creative produce of that period: Is there a deeper spiritual challenge going on and is this now reflected in our era?

To return to Chrétien's account: What are we to make of Perceval, as portrayed in his poem and beyond my initial remarks?

The synopsis is relatively undescriptive, except maybe for some colour references, specifically white and red, with their metallic reflections of silver and gold. This is understandable, as it is a poem that would have its own means of expression that could be lost in translation to prose, as well as being verbally – and theatrically – delivered. Chrétien's writing is otherwise generally well considered by others. The colours have an alchemical ring about them, to which I will return. Additionally, it describes only a golden Grail as a serving dish in the central scene, although the gold description is also distinctly alchemical; it is not referred to as *holy* and a lance that appears may be equally significant. The is an absence of clear reference to a *lance* or *spear* in the movie *Excalibur*, except indirectly as in lightening emanating from the dragon (an oblique reference to the Nordic god *Thor* possibly…); use in conflict or battle (particularly Mordred's spearing of Arthur); Arthur's wounding, or possibly in the name *Lancelot* (unlikely etymologically, but…) has troubled me. The presence of women in Chrétien is also now notable, in varied and erotic contexts, even to one carrying the Grail in what will now be referred to as a *procession*. But what to make of this feature?

There are themes and images that can be comfortably taken into the Christian context, such as the bleeding lance, the *graal* (alt. spelling) as a cup, the host that sustains the wounded King and more. But, equally easily, and maybe with the other emphases I will come to, these could be placed in a more Celtic or broader Pagan context.

For example, the bleeding lance as a symbol of wounding and blood revenge, or alternatively as a sexual reference, including the wounding of the Fisher King. The *graal* as a dish or bowl with the platter could be food and drink, the never-ending supply of which is replete in Pagan mythology, not only as a source of nourishment, but also rejuvenation, so touching on the *healing* theme that I want to emphasise. The host as sustenance for the wounded Fisher King appears more Christian and is confined to the last problematic paragraph.

Not that I am ignoring this healing theme in Christianity, it is just that the *host* as sustenance is maintaining, but not healing the wounded King; it is Perceval's attention to answering of the Grail question that will do this. I find this differentiation significant. The painful wound is identified as a javelin (a Celtic word for a spear) through the thighs, which is really a euphemism for a genital or sexual injury; this puts a different emphasis on the bleeding lance as a symbol of the wound, and the procession maybe as a ritual of healing. It also resonates with the three drops of blood in the snow that reminds Perceval of his beloved Blancheflor elsewhere in the poem and reinforces at least the erotic, if not sexual associations.

Of further interest is that Perceval's silence does not just involve the Grail, but "not asking why the lance bled or what is done with the grail or who was being served by the grail and silver platter". This is far more expansive than the limited understanding that has otherwise found its way down the years. Of course, these all fundamentally relate to the Fisher King and his wounding, although I have hinted about other aspects in the Celtic world, as well as matters sexual. There is more here than meets the eye and, of course, the Church would like to have none of the sexual aspects and limit any healing to Jesus via the Grail as chalice. The Christian agenda is fairly straightforward, too obviously so maybe.

Overall, the actual procession is very ceremonial; it is a ritual and in this context, a ritual of healing, for a wound that is possibly sexual in nature. The answering of the Grail question is its culmination, and it is being asked of the naïve Perceval, an innocent (a further Christian reference). He is also maybe a virgin, the nights with Blancheflor notwithstanding: He is certainly psychologically – and inevitably given his circumstances – tied to his mother; which, interestingly, is announced at the conclusion of the ritual after the girl in mourning admonishes him for failing to ask the question. The later further admonishment by a rather deliberately repulsive woman reinforces his failure. It also juxtaposes the young girl with a hag; quite a Celtic theme of the varying faces of the feminine and a common challenge – with sexual overtones – to knights on mythological quests.

The feminine element is strong and continuous, as is the relative emphasis on youth and beauty. As well as the girl and lady immediately above, the Grail and platter – sources of nourishment and maybe healing – are carried by girls; there is also the girl who prophesies and sets in motion the vengeance theme with Kay's act of violence. It is also she that is carrying the magic potential, it seems, and indirectly the power. This is associated with a jester's involvement; he proves to be prophetic, so he is more likely a bard or magician in the guise of a shamanic trickster. The scene of Blancheflor adds another dimension to the story, that of love. Another scene with the woman in the tent shows his lack of knowledge and initiation in matters sexual with his misinterpretation and reliance on his mother's education. However, such seemingly chance or inept encounters often contain a truth either directly or revealed later in the poem. This may indicate a psychological wisdom that one's errors and trauma may also be a path to salvation.

Then there is Perceval's mother, whose fainting he forgets and whose death would be seen as related to his leaving. Although it is psychologically necessary that mother 'dies' in the development in a youth's initiatory transition to manhood, it is also related to trauma and wounding of its own kind. The psychological wisdom here is that the various aspects of 'innocence' that Perceval displays are associated with a lack of maturity, brought about by a failure of initiation in the 'growing up' sense; also, it is important to note that he had an absent father. Perceval's *forgetting* recalls for me the binary of forgetting:remembering that was explored in Part One and its relationship to trauma; I will go no further with it here, although it hovers elsewhere in the poem.

If Perceval is the Welsh Peredur, he has come up before in Part One, as the King in Wales who Merlin fights with at the battle of Arthuret. He appeared there to lose three brothers, although it is not entirely clear whose brothers these are. However, here we have him having lost his father and two brothers as well as the battle association, and one reason why he is raised by his mother in isolation. The grief that surrounds Merlin would seem to be from the same source as that which afflicts Perceval's mother; maybe this is more than a coincidence. I would briefly mention that Arthur is in Carlisle and also Caerleon later; the two areas that still contend for him – and Merlin – historically; an interesting parallel. Also, isn't "Gawain offers to go to watch how Perceval behaves and to bring him back through more diplomatic means" strangely reminiscent of the attempt to bring Merlin back from the forest to court in Geoffrey's *Vita*? These connections of and similarities between Merlin and Perceval are tantalising.

Reference has been made to the rather distinct and different tone in the last paragraph in the poem about Perceval. Up until this point, I had seen the Fisher King as being the man fishing at the beginning synonymous with the wounded man who is the focus of the procession and all it entails. Yet in this later paragraph the two appear to become father and son, as well as being closely related by blood to Perceval. This seems to obfuscate and even contradict what precedes it, but this can also be seen to be something engaged with if the poem is compared to Geoffrey's *Vita* and the earlier reference to Perceval's father and brothers. It is almost as if there is a pattern here that may represent bloodlines and families closely knit around these events, at least in fable. Blood across this spectrum of meanings gives it a deeply symbolic relevance.

All in all, I find that whilst the themes might be ambivalent in their religious and cultural form from a modern perspective looking back, but if read in the context of the time there is – by comparison to Geoffrey – only a slight Christian gloss. One only has to read the paragraph about Perceval's encounters with Blancheflor to see how non-Christian the poem is, although I would suggest that if sexual consummation did not occur, it was not for Christian reasons. More dominant are the Celtic themes that can be easily misinterpreted to suit the desires of the interpreter, instead of seeing them in their traditional, historical, ancestral, mythological, magical and archetypal context.

With that adjectival overload to emphasise the point, it is time to move on. There is more in the poem, were I to take a critical and academic position, but which I am not. I have also gone into some depth about the Grail specifically as well as with other topics, such as the feminine and sexuality, which I consider important. This is because I want to make Perceval the template, if you like, and include these major themes in a little detail, although more will be forthcoming in the relevant sections that follow this about the other questers. What I am trying to do is extract and elucidate the themes that pertain to this work, rather than entertain academic pretensions, or engage in scholarly argument.

Peredur

At the back of my mind has been the association of Peredur with Merlin at the beginning of Geoffrey's *Vita*. It is worth noting that Geoffrey also mentioned him in his earlier *History* as *Peredurus*, a legendary ruler of Britain, who was the fifth and youngest son born to the similarly legendary *Morvidus*, King of the Britons. It is easy to see how the three sons who died at Arthuret in 573 could be Peredur's brothers. This is reinforced elsewhere where I read, "Peredur inherits his father's lands in the north after his father and brothers die in battle," in one of many synopses of Peredur available online.

There are simply too many rabbit holes beckoning here, so I will stay on the surface and comment that in my broad research it is relatively obvious that the history being drawn on, which includes these various personages, is late in the 6thC. This is where Geoffrey locates Merlin as well as Peredur in *Vita*. It seems to me that this significant period is drawn upon for many stories, poems and is the stuff of legend. For the purpose of this account, the earlier 5thC post-Roman period that includes Vortigern and his dealings with the Anglo-Saxons, which has a very Romanesque British flavour about it, and is located in the more southern region that envelops the more mythic layer of Merlin. Although vying second in this account, it has taken premier and almost exclusive status in the modern imagination.

I am left with two temporarily separated, but otherwise interrelated periods that resonate with each other; the mythic one of South Wales together with the English West Country (hence including Glastonbury) in the South, and the more historical and legendary one of North Welsh, Scottish and English kingdoms in the North. I am further left with little doubt that the latter is the source of Geoffrey's necessity to write *Vita*, as well as

Chrétien's ensuing *Perceval* that contains – for the first documented time – the Grail legend as we know it today. I have eschewed going forward into the subsequently Christianised accounts of the Grail and Arthurian legends – with the exception of Wolfram's Parzival – preferring, as I did with Geoffrey, to look back and see that where Chrétien derived his story is elsewhere apart from his own imagination, and also being one reason that, somewhat like Geoffrey with Merlin in *Vita*, I earlier provided the Perceval story in some detail.

Before I progress, I would just like to mention something I noticed about Peredur's name. I have always been troubled by the names Uther and Arthur being admixed with more Roman ones, including Uther's brother, Aurelius Ambrosius. I also made earlier comment about -*thur* in relation to the Norse god, Thor. The syllable -*dur* could also easily be written as -*thur* because in Old English (the term for describing the language used in this Anglo-Saxon historical period) the letter *d* with a cross represents *th*. Is Perdur in fact Arthur and not Merlin? The plot thickens.

There are many summaries of Peredur; this one is an abbreviated version that covers the main points relevant to my inquiry, taken from BBC Wales online:

> *Similar to Chrétien de Troyes' romance Perceval, the Story of the Grail, Peredur son of Efrawg is one of the three Welsh romances associated with the Mabinogion.*
>
> *The story survives in both the White Book of Rhydderch and the Red Book of Hergest, sources of the tales of the Mabinogion, and tells the life-story of Peredur.*
>
> *It is likely Peredur was a Brythonic (a branch of the Celts) prince ruling over a region in Northern England. He has a father, Efrawg, believed to be*

etymologically linked to York.

Efrawg dies when Peredur is young, and his mother raises him in isolation in woods. As he comes of age he meets a group of knights, and goes with them to the court of King Arthur.

At the court he suffers the ridicule of the knight Cei and sets off, promising to reclaim his honour. On his travels he meets two of his uncles. The first shows him how to bear arms, and instructs him not to question the significance of what he sees.

The second uncle reveals a severed head on a platter (a major departure from Chrétien's account that continues henceforth along a differing path).

Peredur continues on his journeys, staying with the nine witches of Gloucester and falling in love with Angharad Golden-Hand.

He returns to Arthur's court, and eventually learns that the severed head was that of his cousin.

The cousin had been killed by the witches of Gloucester. Aggrieved, Peredur avenges his family members, and returns home a hero.

The books mentioned in the text above, along with the renowned *Welsh Triads*, were written subsequent to Chrétien in the 13-14thC period; however, their poetic sources are well established as being much – centuries – earlier. In effect, they provide a kind of parallel text to the ones drawn on to date and, to my mind, connect back to the source material in a more direct and authentic manner.

The brief outline here is so similar to Chrétien that it doesn't bear commenting on, until it arrives at the "severed head on a platter". With the exception of the platter, this is hardly a Grail procession, so I am going to 'pause' that account in Chrétien for the time being and instead see where this outline takes me… because it is starting to feel somewhat familiar. Peredur discovers later that this is the head of his cousin, which makes him related to the Fisher King; in fact, his son in some accounts.

Why Peredur seemingly has not recognised the head as that of his cousin at the time seems odd; it is also worth noting there is no issue about questioning here in this more Pagan material. This makes me *question* whether Peredur actually did recognise the head, but stayed silent; was it culturally appropriate in some way to take this stance? This puts a different light on the questioning issue in Chrétien and Wolfram, where there is *guilt* associated with the apparent failure, either somewhat psychoanalytically about his mother, or more psychospiritually because the King and hence the Land are not healed as a consequence. The morality of this issue remains unclear to me, although it makes me wonder whether Perceval was appropriate in *not* asking the supposed question.

I am immediately reminded of John the Baptist, with the severed head on a platter, and will return to this imagery later when the Grail is looked at in more detail, as well as when the connections to the Crucifixion story are explored. However, and more immediately significant in spite of the above cousin reference, is the strong association with *Brân the Blessed*, who is a king in Welsh mythology, with a name that is considered to mean a *crow* or *raven*:

> He (Brân) hid himself in the bodies of the fallen Irish.
> When the cauldron attendants came along and threw
> him in, he spread his body out in all directions,
> shattering the cauldron but sacrificing himself in the

process. During the great fight Brân took a fatal blow to the foot, and as he lay in his deathbed he gave his men these last instructions: "Cut my head off and take it to London. Eventually you must bury it in the state on the White Hill of London (thought to be the White Tower location in the Tower of London), turning my head towards France." Ceremonially they cut off Brân's head and left Ireland. (From Branwen ferch Llŷr).

According to the Welsh Triads, Brân's head was buried in London... As long as it remained there, Britain would be safe from invasion. However, King Arthur dug up the head, declaring the country would be protected only by his great strength.

(Both quotes from Wikipedia, slightly modified)

The associations in the above go deep into Welsh and British pre-history and will be left at this point, except where they link to the present inquiry, both here and forthcoming. Arthur's presence is worthy of note, linking him to this era and its mythology, indicating his presence to be fundamentally mythological, to my way of thinking, both here and elsewhere.

Almost in passing – because these associations seem to be piling up – the *White Book of Rhydderch* is valuable Welsh source material and is named after *Rhydderch Hael*, a king who flourished in the Brittonic kingdom of *Alt Clut*, or Strathclyde in the late 6thC, and who is obviously now the Rhydderch of Geoffrey's *Vita*. This seems to me particularly so because *hael* can mean *generous*, and there is a generosity of spirit shown by Rhydderch in *Vita*. Although not directly present in the name, I am drawn to the phonetic association of hael with *hale*, as in 'hale and hearty' and thus with *healing* and *wholeness*.

As earlier indicated, healing is a theme that interests me personally, but is also one that I feel languishes in the research around the accounts that I have related to date. This may be reinforced by the nominated books as being *red* and *white*, which is by now a familiar alchemical theme, present with the mythic dragons and weaving their way through to the medieval houses of Lancaster and York with their regal aspirations, to become further reinforced in Chrétien's poetry.

Finally, to the witches: Who are they? There is ambiguity here in that Peredur stays with them, yet later avenges his family's loss by – presumably – killing them. Gloucester locates them in the southern region of the inquiry, relatively close to Glastonbury, which is a contender for the title of Avalon where Arthur was conveyed after his final battle for healing. This was in the company of women from Avalon, who were also responsible for this healing. There is at least an association here with the feminine, wounding, healing and the Grail that supports the procession and other features. Yet however enticing these associations are, they remain just that.

I believe there are two areas here that written history has obfuscated. The first is the now familiar Christianisation of the Grail legends and all that surrounds it, being primarily the Celtic Tradition, and then subsequently associated with the Passion. The second is related, and is how women are perceived in this era now under a Christian yoke. There are ambiguities and ambivalences aplenty, which all makes me feel there is an attempt to gloss the feminine with a relative demonisation in such naming as *witches*, unless conforming to the pure and innocent feminine picture otherwise presented. I find this to be a contrast with those women who are healers and work with death and dying.

Celtic women are of a different nature than the one generally portrayed here. They are more powerful, sexually autonomous and carried functions like magic and healing in their communities; no wonder Christianity then felt – and still feels – threatened by the feminine. In addition, they are clearly associated with mythological tradition, including the Tuatha Dé Danann and the various other civilisations of Britain and Ireland prior to history. In imaginative terms, the feminine has retreated elsewhere to become *Faery*. It is my contention that this is one way to approach the feminine in this borderline between history and myth; it could be equated with the Jungian unconscious and specifically the archetypal *anima*; the feminine that resides – known or unknown – within us all and not exclusively men, in deference to the Jungian position on the anima.

Yet Faery is not just a term for the subjective unconscious feminine. There is the Celtic belief here that the previous occupants of these Isles retreated into the Land when conquered. The Tuatha represent a more objective state – altered maybe – of consciousness that visits us in liminal states and dreaming. Here we are in the realms of mythic beings and folklore, such as *elves* and *dwarves*, where concepts like *changeling* are accepted as real by those who have faith. There is often a sexual quality to the interchanges between Faery and the realm of the present human occupants, even to the production of children. Here, Merlin is a notable example; the supposed product of an elf and human woman. Of course, the Christian position is to demonise these dimensions, such that they become *incubi* and *succubi* and Merlin's father now becomes the Devil himself.

I am reminded of the Norse legends here and the complex role female figures play, including the *Valkyries* and their function with the dead after battle, as well as the *Norns* who weave and govern *wyrd*, or fate. I have made association to Norse and associated mythology elsewhere and how it permeates and influences these tales in sometimes subtle ways. This is hardly a surprise when their proximity of location is considered, particularly with their contacts in northern Britain that were contemporaneous with the Anglo-Saxon invasions-cum-migrations after the Romans departed, and the background to the more mythic elements in this inquiry.

I have followed up some of the leads indicated, including those related to Odin/Woden and Loki. I believe they are significant and have no difficulty in seeing these mythic tales both overlapping and permeating the ones under examination here. To see the story of the Grail as exclusively Celtic is simplistic, although I have tended to favour that common terminology for ease of communication. It is also why I see that an appreciation of Germanic mythology, legend and history is important in filling in some – maybe many – of the apparent gaps that this study presents. Of course, this will never be completed in the cognitive sense, but this inquiry is an attempt to come to peace with it – heal, if you like – in terms of my own life story.

Parzival

The figure of Parzival intrigues me; by this time early in the 13thC the Christianisation is readily apparent in Wolfram von Eschenbach's poem, although the sources and intent behind it is unclear. Written in Middle High German, it is effectively a continuation of Chrétien's *Perceval* and follows a similar pattern, including the legend of the Grail. However, it is a departure from other continuations with some distinctive language, particularly with the names, as well as using an indirect alchemical nomenclature and a quite different image of the Grail to how it is presently conceived.

The various Grail poets are directly or indirectly accused of philosophical and scientific naïvité amongst other rather modern scholarly judgements, indicating these works somehow represent an earlier and immature stage of our human development. Whilst reading Chrétien, I was impressed about the psychological wisdom and its subtle expression. I believe this to be present in Wolfram along with humour and sarcasm that reaches the satirical, in my opinion. The subtlety around the Grail procession, use of symbolism and spiritually scientific – not pre-scientific –alchemical wisdom, I find unrecognised or unacknowledged.

Whilst looking for a suitable synopsis, I found it intriguing that most modern commentators provide much in the way of detail about the various people and acts involved, but fail to provide the depth and richness that Wolfram provides. Here, in one near 600-word online synopsis, is the relevant comment on these aspects. As the core of the story is the Grail, the seeker and healing, the absence of this is notable; maybe the modern sensibility finds such content just too difficult to reconcile:

> *Parzival finds lodging at Munsalvaesche one night, where he sees the mysteries surrounding the Grâl, but he fails to free Anfortas by asking the Question; when he leaves the next day, he encounters Sigune, who chides him for failing to ask the Question.*

And…

> *Feirefiz accompanies Parzival to Munsalvaesche, where Parzival frees Anfortas from his suffering by asking the Question.*

Wolfram's work is complex and subtle, though largely following Chrétien's romance, such that this could be seen as a continuation; but it is more colourful and quite different in tone. As Chrétien is more ritualistic and magical, there is an air of ceremony and mystery in Wolfram, with the sense of the unknown impinging in the work in a mystical manner that is often difficult to grasp.

Instead of being lazy and trying to find a suitable synopsis, it may be easier to let the work stand as a whole and make relevant comment about it. Instead, I will simply provide an account for comparison; although, unlike with Chrétien, I will reserve the core of the poem for elucidation later when examining the central experience of Parzival in the castle of the Grail King, Anfortas.

The play of words, particularly in the names of people and places, is unique. There is some direct copying, such as with the figure of Gahmuret, although in general it is idiosyncratically Wolfram. For example, Herzeloyde may mean 'heart's sorrow' and Sigune something like 'embraced' in Middle High German; interestingly in Norse mythology, the similar Sigyn is 'victorious girl-friend'. Although a little tangential, Sig is the root of *Sigel* that is a rune for the Sun; I suspect further runic associations in the names. The sorceress, Cundrie, is a hag who presents a more overtly Celtic image, whose name has both sexual and runic associations, in my opinion. Wolfram's use of double entendres, often with a risqué component, is readily apparent and often avoided in any commentary. There is a lot of associated humour and vague and indirect reference to sexuality; women are paid strong and healthy attention. Grammatically and phonetically the poem is often ambiguous, which is how it also seems to end, maybe deliberately so.

Parzival is presented as an aspiring king, who is ignorant of this fact and living outside of society. In his development various initiatory stages can be identified and he is put through both literal and symbolic tests to become the king. His literal self-wounding with his hands drawing blood mimics the bleeding lance and therefore identifies him closely with the Grail procession. The various central characters are closely related in a familial manner and reinforce the bloodline aspect of the Grail, at least as a background theme.

In summary to this point, the details of the procession and the various symbols in Wolfram are more detailed and richer than anyone else to date, prior to the Grail going down the Christian path in a more exclusive manner, as initiated by Robert de Boron. What is significant is that the Grail and lance are given equal importance, and the Grail itself is portrayed as a precious stone with magical power. As in Chrétien, it is not associated with the *Passion*, where this term refers to both the Last Supper, Crucifixion and other events around that time in Jesus' storyline.

In general, here and elsewhere Wolfram appears to complete Chrétien's work. Wolfram gives a name to most characters and expands on the family relationships, such that a clearer image of the Grail Family and bloodline emerge. In addition to the nature of the Grail, a significant and probable alchemical feature, Wolfram also introduces the Middle East to his poem. This is with Parzival's half-brother and other features, such as the apparent play on black and white and the attempt at unification including East and West in a literal manner (and possibly a reference to the Crusades), as well as further symbolic alchemical reference.

In fact, the healing motif, as in Anfortas' wound and its treatment, is pre-eminent and strong, which brings me to the question the Grail Seeker has to ask to effect the wound healing in Parzival. The question itself has changed from being about the Grail and what it serves, to asking directly of the wounded King what *ails* him. In other words, it is not a philosophical or even mystical enquiry, it is about healing. Once asked, the King is healed. Further reflection on the question will be left to the more detailed examination of the Grail.

I find this point very significant. In my experience dreams provide information, but it is up to us to consciously act on this with choices, decisions etc. There is a parallel here in that the various icons in the procession scene provide symbolic information that sustains the King, but does not heal him; it is Parzival's task to understand what he is seeing, beyond whatever it is that has inhibited this process on his first visit to the Grail castle, and act by asking the relevant question. There is a direct parallel here with my dream process.

There is much about Wolfram to like and further material to expand on, maybe a future task… But at this point, I would like to return to my own story to see how it compares – if at all – to this section on the Grail Seeker.

Osman

The title of this section refers to my spiritual name derived from the runes and other psychic experiences. I use it selectively in my spiritual activities and with others in our community. I am using it here as an identity in this inquiry, which is beginning to mirror Parzival in many ways.

I would like to share a significant dream that followed my rather abrupt departure from medical practice, when I was unsure about where my direction would be from that point. The decision to leave, although fatefully inevitable and by choice irrevocable, had been made without consideration for what my next career and professional move might be, if at all.

This is the third dream of mine that will be presented here; I intend it be the last, unless the gods provoke my prophetic propensity and confer more before this work is completed:

I see a man, as if crucified. He has a stake, like a huge silver needle, driven through his testicles from in front, like a giant pin. The pain is transmitted via hammer blows to this by an identifiable but unknown male figure. This stake passes through him into the side of a building, from which he is suspended by his arms that are tethered together behind his back and thus painfully stretched above him with his suspension. It looks more like a torture scene; he is being publicly 'crucified' in this manner on the upper outside part of an old medieval building that is part of a continuous row of houses, like an English village or town street.

The man is nearly or recently expired. Whether the pain keeps him alive is unclear, but there is little, if any, physical response. He then begins to naturally fall from his tethering onto an animal, maybe an ass, and onto its back. Nobody stops this and the ass moves off and at a neighbouring building, maybe that of a 'Witch', where white fluid, like milk, is poured over the body by her. Again, it is unclear whether this will revive or embalm him.

(Sacrificial Dream, 2014)

Surprisingly I had not, until recently, given the above dream the kind of attention that the Original Dream has received after I had it. I had maybe *forgotten* it, or failed to ask the *question*.

This dream, following on from the end of my career in medical practice, was during a turbulent period in all aspects of my life, personal and professional, which goes partway to explaining this ignoring, but not entirely; *forgetfulness* is obviously involved. I have always had the sense that it would connect to the other dreams when I looked at it, and that I needed to do this at an appropriate time; although this is not to say that the images themselves did not have an intervening effect on me, irrespective of my conscious stance.

Immediately identifying the image as a crucifixion may relate more to how I was experiencing my circumstances at the time, although the mythic significance has not escaped me, particularly now as I address the Grail further. It is as if the word *crucifixion* defines what is happening, whereas the actual scene is more like a public torture; I am unsure as to whether it is actually an intended execution though, because of the lack of clarity at the end. Also, because if it were, say, an execution in the style of hanging, drawing and quartering, then it is really only the first of these stages. Beheading is not present and, although often a component of drawing and quartering, castration is only implied. There is something quite ritualistic and possibly initiatory about it, as there often is in executions anyway.

The crucifixion impression is enhanced by such features as impaling, although this could refer more to the wound of the Fisher King and inferred in *Excalibur's* Arthur, who somewhat 'doubles' as the Fisher King. Any association to Jesus' story is augmented by the animal that carries him, an ass, as in Palm Sunday prior to the events of the Crucifixion in the Passion. This is all very dense imagery, overlapping not only the Crucifixion, but the Grail King's wounding. Yet there is more: I have referred to the lance elsewhere, as in Arthur's final wounding that led to a similarly indeterminate state of alive:dead (there is more to be said about this dyad, it is also a component of the Great Cycle of Existence, after all). Also, the lance features prominently here and more distinctly as a tool of pain, wounding and suffering.

The lance is one of the *hallows* of the Tuatha, it may be recalled, and this will be returned to. Here, my attention is drawn to the image that flows between all three dreams; being the metallic pointed pylon, the cut-off fountain, and now the pin that is driven through the man's testicles. The lance was also used by the Roman centurion in the Crucifixion myth to pierce the side of Jesus, from which blood then flowed and was collected in a vessel, supposedly the chalice of the Last Supper; it must be remembered that these are all later accretions to the core Crucifixion account as conveyed in the Synoptic Gospels. Interestingly, if I were to make what is called a *bindrune* of the initials of my present name (when the runes for each letter are combined into one glyph, and considered of magical import), the resulting image is like a lance or sword and resembles the outline of a pylon. With the lance, we are back in Grail territory, particularly as the dream itself is set in a medieval village or town. These interconnections in the dreams, as well as between the dreams, movie and Charm, will continue to be explored as I move more extensively into the Grail legends.

But before doing this, it will serve to look more fully at the second segment of the dream and how these images relate. Reference has already been made to the ass and Palm Sunday. Maybe, more significantly, is the image in *Excalibur* when Perceval is on the Quest and sees Gawain emerge from a forest strapped to the back of a horse in a supine position with his throat cut. He is dead. "The man is nearly or recently expired" reinforces the liminal space he is in with respect to life:death or the Great Cycle, as in the torture scene itself, but does raise the question as to whether he can be revived or resurrected, with the ongoing Christian association of this literal inquiry. This indeterminant state takes him to the woman, where embalming is also presented as an option.

The white fluid is poured; I do not recall seeing a vessel in the dream, but one is clearly implied by this action. More ambiguity rests with the white fluid. In the context of the dream, this could be an herb or drug mixture to effect the "revive or embalm" options, or possibly as pain relief and a healing tool. I do identify her as a Witch, which is a little enigmatic; at this stage, pointing to the theme of healing and the role of the feminine, with a backdrop of how such women were viewed from the conventional religious perspective. After all, she could be working counter to the desires of the torturer; somehow be in league with him, or even working together in some ritualistic pattern This is not clear either then or now. A little tangentially, white as a colour reminds me of the feminine in alchemy, as well as the white dragon and its associations.

Of course, a more psychological interpretation is also available. The white fluid could obviously be breast milk or semen. Again, it is ambiguous, unclear, and presenting itself now to be disentangled. Although inferred, these possibilities do 'fit the bill' at many levels and are worth exploring, particularly in the case of any personal and shadow dynamics related to trauma. In fact, the whole dream could be seen in this reductive light, which could be valuable, but I contend not all of the picture. There is also the implied vessel that takes the imagery back to the Original Dream (the jar and needing a vice to open it), as well as the visionary tale that the youthful Merlin tells Vortigern of the dragons below the lake, which also have many of the associations outlined immediately above.

Apart from the unidentified victim who, rather like the Original Man, feels more like *me* than the others, there are two other figures. The man who is hammering is identifiable; I see him, but he always stays peripheral. As I write now, I have the urge to see the hammer as identifying him with the Norse god *Thor*. There are several reasons for this, without going into the mythic background of the god himself. The first is that he is identified by his hammer, called *Mjölnir*, with its ambivalent function as a weapon and its capacity to heal, as well as to confer blessings; it is often used protectively as a talisman. I mention these facts to bring the Scandinavian worldview into the picture again, but also because the hammer and hammering reinforces the deep ambivalence that is present throughout the dream.

I have always been impressed by some of the disparity in the various names that are drawn from the time of Merlin and Arthur, including these figures themselves. Arthur's father is Uther, which strikes me as a very chthonic name when compared to his brother and prior King, Aurelius Ambrosius, which is distinctly more Romano-British. Maybe we have simply placed too much emphasis on names, as evidenced by the various explanations of Merlin's name in this regard? Arthur is considered Brythonic, or from a branch of the Celtic language that relates to Wales and other territories. It supposedly means *bear*, but has this word other connotations, including astrological and shamanic? Or, quite tangentially, is the *thur* part, that is after all common to Uther, related to Thor? This reasoning is intuitive and not backed academically, to my knowledge, but it marks another level of connection with the Norse world and its mythology with the Celtic. The lifting of the massive Mjölnir and the drawing of the sword from the stone do have parallels.

However, I have noticed that I am not alone in this line of inquiry. I also believe we get too weighed down by etymology and lapse into a restricted scientific and cognitive way of looking at these issues. Phonetics can also have a part to play, more so because we don't have clear access to how languages like Old English and Old Norse were actually spoken. So, here's another one: What if the commonly used *All Father* description of the Norse Odin becomes *Arthur*? Because phonetically across language differences, it actually does. Arthur certainly has such qualities and now blurs the boundaries with Merlin, as *Woden*. I'll stop there; it's fun, but inconclusive… though highly suggestive.

I also do not intend to go into these connections beyond where they relate to the present inquiry; it is simply too vast. But I do want to stress that these relationships between peoples that preceded the Roman invasion and run a parallel course behind and beyond it, occupying the first millennium until the invasion of the Normans that itself still had a Norse connection, are more significant than we have given credit to. The Irish *Book of Invasions* testifies to this, and the Tuatha will be returned to. Similar acknowledgement should be given the Germanic peoples, and particularly the Norse, and not simply focus on the restricted and presently distorted picture of the Viking that, after all, was really only in the period 800 – 1100 CE. Seafaring peoples and their movements have largely dictated pre- and early history, more so than we have given credit to.

The Witch is another figure who can be rewardingly explored in the Norse worldview, which I have indicated earlier. Is she rescuing the victim, or part of the process? Is this process ritualistic, initiatory, even shamanic, and designed – like the Crucifixion – as a process of deep transformation? Maybe this will all only become clearer as the feminine unfolds, because it is all too easy to see her in a dark light (paradoxical metaphor deliberate).

I would like to put myself in the position of a Grail Seeker; the emphasis is on *a* rather than *the*; in effect, and for reasons that will become apparent, I consider that we are potentially all of us Grail Seekers.

At the beginning of the previous section, I recounted the first part of the Original Dream to kind of set the tone for what follows. I will be returning to it later with an expanded elucidation of the literal and symbolic Grail, but now want to focus on the Sacrificial Dream, above, along with the second half of the Original Dream:

I'm now in the countryside of the island working
as a doctor. Julie, my receptionist, takes the patients'

cards from the cupboard. There are two; the 'original' man and woman. I have seen the woman before, but not the man, although I have treated his son. The man enters, emerging from a mist. He wears a jacket and white polo-neck sweater; he is worn out, exhausted. I look in the cupboard where there is a jar, I realise I may need to use a vice to open it.

There is a resonance here between the original man and the Grail or Fisher King in my opinion, maybe more so now than with any of the extended associations I have already given, when looking at this dream earlier in Part One. He is smartly attired and the sweater is a distinct feature, giving him a debonaire, if not a distinctly regal appearance. The polo-neck gives me the impression of a priest, as well. These associations are more Celtic, as is his emergence from a mist, yet in a modern guise and context.

What reinforces the wounded Fisher King image is the fact that he is "worn out, exhausted". He is presenting to me for treatment, as he has an appointment via the feminine in Julie. The cupboard is an area for storage and where the patient cards are kept, which reinforces his purpose in emerging from the mist for my attention. It is as if he is coming from the Otherworld; I wonder if he has been neglected and deprived, and have we done this to the world he comes from? In helping him, would I also be rehabilitating the world he comes from; that is, am I healing both? This potential regarding the Otherworld, or the Land, is reinforced by this taking place in the countryside of the island. Further, is the island itself related to Avalon?

My feeling is that the jar is associated with his treatment, although this is not entirely clear; it certainly resonates with some historical images of the Grail. The vice is an ambiguous and enigmatic image already discussed, but the issue here is that I don't resolve that ambiguity, nor do I then open it. In a way, this could equate to my not addressing and solving the riddle; in effect *not asking the question*. Instead, I focussed on the first part of the dream, as encouraged by my analyst and her preference, and left the second part unresolved. In doing so, the man – effectively the Celtic priest-king aspect of myself – is left unhealed.

There may – may – be a further association with the vice that has just come to me. Given that I am now associating this with a failure to ask questions, which any good doctor would do, I wonder whether the vice may also refer to a lack of *voice*. I did not ask the man why he is here, what his problem is (what are his *symptoms* and what is then my *diagnosis*) and how I can help him. These are locked up, in a way, and I have not addressed them. Instead, I half-glorify in having had a classical Jungian *self* dream to kick off my analysis and charge back into medical practice and continue my cavalier lifestyle; yet I have not accessed the power, connected with my soul, or realised that what I am re-engaging with is a *wasteland*.

In 2014 and more than I suspect, my direction was now a void and my life more precarious than I had hitherto reckoned with. Instead of paying due heed to the dream, I tried a resurrection based on my prior abilities and talents to then witness them successively fail, in spite of my best application and – what I considered at the time – pure *intent*. In 2020, immediately prior to the pandemic, I pushed myself beyond the physical limits and surrendered, I started to realise that my heart was more important than my head, when it 'told' me so; physical manifestations can do that, but it is important to catch their symbolic message before a fear-ridden medical diagnosis intervenes. I went into an isolated forest den for a year to retreat and reassess. During this time and immediately afterwards, my attention was drawn to Merlin… or, maybe more correctly, he was drawing my attention to him. This account is the outcome of that relationship and in it I am addressing the questions that I have failed to ask. Because, again in the Sacrificial Dream, I have not asked the necessary question.

But I am answering it now…

My life has been religiously governed by Church of England Christianity. The impact on my family during childhood was mainly around the holiday occasions of Easter and Christmas within social settings, and some other interesting times, such as a Church ceremony at Harvest Festival… although we did say Grace before meals. Interestingly, this latter time was also that of the Gaelic Lugnasa(dh), one of the four reputed seasonal festival times from Celtic traditions that were interspersed through the year. The other festivals are Imbolc, Beltane and Samhain, all of which have some sort of Christian appropriation, possibly with the exception of Beltane; simply too raunchy with its deeper and more orgiastic connotations.

When isolated from family at boarding school in adolescence, I started to experience some solace with the religious services, being ornate and theatrical in the High Church, and I subsequently underwent Confirmation. The emotion I experienced in the services confused me, although I enjoyed the experience. With an option to further this interest, I studied Saint Mark (one of the Synoptic Gospels, and maybe the foundation of the others) with a tutor who was a Doctor of Divinity. However, when he failed to satisfy my curiosity that Mark's Gospel after the Crucifixion may not have been written by Mark, so questioning for me the validity of the Resurrection, I put religion in the bin and proceeded with a scientific career. Analysis changed all this.

What I had come to realise was that Christianity in Britain had and still has a distinct gloss and that the Pagan elements showed through, if one cared to look for them. Once my more heathen outlook was uncovered in my therapeutic analysis, I went looking further. Ultimately Druidry was the umbrella that I believed most satisfied my values; not that of modern revivalism, but the more traditional and shamanistic version, warts and all. Yet somehow I had to reconcile this ancestral affiliation with my personal history: Ultimately, this inquiry took me to Arthur, Merlin and the Grail. This present work can be viewed as my offering to such a reconciliation. Even though I seem to favour a Pagan outlook, in the Grail and figures within the legends there is a mystical and magical trend that I find continuity with, such that I do not now experience any psychic division. As this narrative moves on from here, I trust this will become more apparent.

To compare the torture of the man as a crucifixion seems strange to me now, yet it was how I reported the dream then, although the imagery is not compatible except as a hanging through the hands being somehow tethered. Otherwise, it is a painful suspension and inducing suffering. Although it may also have been a manner of crucifying someone historically, I am inclined to see it now as more a torture mechanism, especially with arms being tethered behind and up. I notice my description at the time tends toward 'torture' as the dream progresses. The man is making no sound though and intuitively reminds me of the man of the Original Dream. Of course, he is also related to the wounded Fisher King, a fact I did not know at the time was that the wound itself is similarly afflicted, according to (at least) Chrétien's Perceval.

In spite of my earlier retraction, his being on the back of an ass is a relatively obvious image relatable to Palm Sunday, so giving this a Christian background is not inappropriate. In fact, from a sympathetic magic perspective, it seems valid that Christianity would be crucifying Paganism – which effectively it has done – using the tools inflicted upon its supposed Founder.

Is the torture a way of murdering any responsibility for what the Church has done in its appropriation – including that of the Grail legends themselves – and does it feel guilty? By leaving Jesus on the cross, as Mark did and Christianity still does by honouring the Crucifixion but minimising the Resurrection, does the Church feel responsible and try to make reparation with others, such as Galahad? It's a psychological mess.

Where this dream departs from the earlier one is that it is not I and my jar that is called upon to complete the process, it is a *Witch*. I cannot describe her clearly, though I don't recall her being either a hag or beautiful. I could associate her with Julie, but that does not feel right: She feels 'other'. Yet she has the jar open – if continuation from the earlier dream is valid – something I had not done, and is now using it to treat or heal him. What an irony; the feminine, and a Pagan at that, healing the King (viz. the Saviour) with her skills and potion. I have invoked her here; was I to have recognised that at the time, my life may have taken a different course.

Instead, I failed to ask the questions I am asking now. Unlike Perceval, maybe I needed to fail twice before I got the message; he may have been naïve, but I am a slow learner it seems.

The Passion in Perspective

Preamble

Although I am focusing mainly on the Crucifixion in response to the demands of my dreams, there will be times when the Last Supper and particularly the Resurrection come into the inquiry, so I will make more general use of the term that embraces all these interrelated events: The Passion. I will – and have already – capitalised the terms when they specifically refer to the events in the life of Jesus.

> *"On the Cross Jesus surrendered himself to this Dark Power. He lost everything: friends, disciples, his own people, their law and religion. And at last he had to surrender his God: 'My God, my God, why have you forsaken me.' Even his heavenly Father, every image of a personal God, had to go. He had to enter the Dark Night, to be exposed to the abyss. Only then could he become everything and nothing, opened beyond everything that can be named or spoken; only then could he be one with the darkness, the Void, the Dark Mother who is Love itself..."*

> (Dom Bede Griffiths)

I came across this quote today in my researches, whilst writing this piece and the section that precedes it. I went to it intuitively, because I recalled Dom Bede's view of darkness and the Dark Mother whilst I was doing a little research on dark matter and energy. So, I will head down this rabbit hole for a wee while…

I have been intrigued that the cutting edge of modern physics, in the very large and very small, seems to anticipate changes in our view of ourselves and map onto areas like psychology and medicine. I am, of course, far from alone in this, but it seems extraordinary to me that the whole domain of *energy* is still relatively dismissed in all modern scientific fields; certainly, that has been my professional experience, such that we hold to matter over other non-physical forces and shut ourselves off from avenues that would lead into a more mystical and magical appreciation of our existence. It would also change how we perceive healing. Although we are slowly building on the insights and discoveries of Einstein or others, we still routinely hold to a Newtonian worldview, it seems.

However, at another level of understanding, I should not be surprised. I understand that our physical existence is contained within, and yet continuous with, a far greater non-physical or energetic existence, and that we can appreciate the former through the latter; but the former in and of itself, cannot appreciate the latter. So, when medicine pushes itself to the limits in areas like cancer, it finds more questions, irrationality and ambiguities the more it looks. Unless the discipline leaps into the dark, Dom Bede style, further insights – or *secrets* – will not be revealed. To make such a leap or turnaround would, I contend, lead to the paradigm shift that modern medicine needs to undertake; to see all mental and physical illness and disease in this context is something I routinely do.

This was an understanding I appreciated well over a generation ago whilst practising as a Jungian analyst, when I realised that a branch of physics and mathematics called Chaos Theory was pushing boundaries and describing existence in a manner that was readily translated to Jungian depth psychology (and vice versa). Unfortunately, this particular relationship has not been realised, as yet, and now this theory has lost a lot of its initial lustre. But it did give me insights about how to sort of 'decode' a lot of theories in modern physics. As a brief insightful aside, I wonder how much my earlier appreciation of the life:dead dyad is reflected in Schrödinger's famous mind-game of the cat-in-the-box?

I digress, because it was dark matter and energy that caught my attention this morning and led me to Dom Bede. In simple terms, it seems the current view is that our physical existence comprises only 5% of the mass of the known universe, which exists within an undetectable dark mass of 27% and dark energy of 68%. So let me get whimsical although, in passing, it does somehow reflect Dom Bede's quote.

I have used the term *spiritual* a lot, to date. In some ways, this is in contrast to *religious*, such that religious:spiritual is analogous to exoteric:esoteric or even reality:mysticism. The danger, of course, being that magic cuts across these dyads and makes it quite threatening to religion-as-doctrine, or even medicine-as-science. But I am using the term spiritual, so as not to get too involved in semantics that can prove controversial, such as God, the Divine etc. Yet, if looking at the Trinitarian father, holy ghost and son of the Christian Trinity, spiritual could be analogous to *holy ghost*. There are many moderns who would see spirituality as broader, embracing all three, and compatible in the terms of physics as energy, so implying that matter is a particularly condensed form of energy. Certainly, Einstein sees them as relative and interchangeable and Hiroshima in my dream may be further testament to it.

Take spirit and energy out of the equation, or put it temporarily behind, then we have – according to Freud and my Original Dream – father, mother, son. Maybe this is what Dom

Bede is inferring and the dark matter/energy conundrum points to; even Jung wanted to instate the feminine within the Trinity, so making a quaternary. And recall the Grail legends so far, isn't it littered with fathers and sons, and varied images of the mother, woman or more broadly pictured feminine?

These are simply some speculative thoughts I would like to entertain as I move into the Crucifixion.

The Crucifixion and Resurrection

I have referred to the Sacrificial Dream as a crucifixion; would I have done that were I to have had the dream recently? I don't know, but I now wonder whether I have glossed it with my conditional Christian association of the apparent suffering with the Crucifixion. If I refer back to Mark's Gospel, however, there is no mention at all of pain or suffering, just a simple account of the facts. Also, at that time I would have been conditioned to see the centurion's use of the spear as a part of the story; I hadn't noticed until recently that Mark makes no mention of it: How deep is our conditioning.

When I read Mark now, I feel like I am reading an account of someone going through a ritual process, an initiation. Then again, I would, wouldn't I? Maybe those inclined should get the Bible out, dust it down and read chapters 14-16. And maybe that is why I liken my dream to the Crucifixion, even though the imagery does not directly speak of it. The stages of progress of the man's plight in the dream, the life:death ambiguity and the healing ministrations of the Witch now remind me more of the triple death in its more symbolic representation.

As I read the Sacrificial Dream now, there are far more connections with the wounded Fisher King and his healing. The knowledge that his wound is genital and spear-inflicted, unknown to me consciously at the time of the dream, is remarkably similar. There is little doubt to me now that I am watching the King's wounding – The Fisher King, not the King of the Jews – and healing; although the latter is also being healed and the fact he was also called King now has added significance to me. I am more connected with the imagery in the dream and what is happening, and I ask myself – now – why he is being treated this way, what does it mean?

That the Fisher King's wounding is so readily relatable to that of the Crucifixion story should not surprise me now, nor should it surprise me that some of the poets of the 11-12ᵗʰC would similarly do so and inadvertently play into the hands of the Church's more political motives. De Boron, in particular, by linking the Grail back to the Passion, has provided a momentum that is still sustained in our time. Yet, in my opinion, it is deeply flawed and is making history out of the imagination of some of the men of this time.

Yet in the Grail legends (and in my dream) it is the spear that wounds. And the Grail question is directed toward the person wounded, so as to heal him. In some accounts the spear or the blood that drips from it, is actually used in the healing process; blood is a deep and varied symbol. The Grail is directed toward sustenance, as is the use of the Host, being equivalent to maintenance in medicine, but not actual healing. Any healing involves our active participation in the process as an imperative, a fundamental. In the Eucharist the wafer and wine are a facsimile of the body and blood of Jesus; by a process of sympathetic magic, the receiver then identifies with him. The step I find awkward, is that we are instructed that is because he underwent this process *for* us (and our sins), when it should be a direction *to* us to undergo the same process of initiation and transition. Because this is what the Sacrificial Dream is informing me.

The Church has relatively minimised the Resurrection. I find this strange but not unpredictable, rather like the inversion of responsibility in the Eucharist. By ending the story's emphasis at the Crucifixion, there is an incompleteness of the ritual process of initiation and transformation, and hence healing. My Original Dream stopped here from the healing perspective, whilst the Sacrificial Dream continued it through to the potential of healing. Because now I am asking the questions.

Of interest is that it is Mary Magdalene who first sees Jesus in Mark (or his Gospel continuer at this point); the same Mary "out of whom he had cast seven devils". Although remarkably like a description of a shamanic exorcism, it is the fact that it is Mary who first sees him that intrigues me, rather like it is the Witch who sees the tortured man conveyed by the ass, with the Palm Sunday association. Mary is not stated to have anointed Jesus' feet at the earlier Passover time, but is sometimes so associated; this seems similar to the process the Witch is performing with the tortured man.

"They shall take up serpents; and if they drink any deadly thing, it shall not hurt them; they shall lay hands on the sick, and they shall recover. (Mark 16:18)" are Jesus's final words in Mark, before he was received in heaven. Apart from the first phase resonating with the "breath of the dragon (or serpent)" in the Charm, what is remarkable to me, is the healing emphasis. This caused me to pick up my adolescent Tutor's comment and explore Mark again, specifically Chapter 16 (and more specifically verses 9-20, that are the more questionable ones in terms of authorship). My earlier doubts remain as a consequence, although I can now detect themes that both emphasise the role and importance of women, hence the feminine, and are more distinctly shamanic. One day, I may return here and dig further…

In my opinion, when seen as a whole, the Passion contains many resemblances to the Grail story. It is not difficult to see how Christians would relate the Grail legends to the Passion, as they are harmonically related across time. In Jung's terminology they both derive from an archetypal pattern that is distinctly shamanic and focussed on healing; no wonder I have been drawn to the feminine in so many ways. But this is not the only prior complex of stories that express this archetypal pattern, as examination of Celtic prehistory has revealed. It is just that the story of a distinctly shamanic man two thousand years ago of Middle-Eastern origins has usurped the equivalent stories in our own cultural, traditional and ancestral heritage. But maybe the tide is turning, and Merlin is pointing the way…

This section is left incomplete, if the issue of the lance – now as *Lance*, including the similar descriptions of spear and javelin – is not dealt with: I have chosen to capitalise the lance to Lance to put it on, at least, the same footing as the Grail. What is increasingly apparent in the Grail stories, once they are stripped of their Christian accretions, is that the Lance is more significantly involved than the Grail in the procession, as well as the healing of the wounded Fisher King. It may be apparent that the lessening of emphasis of the Grail is reflected in my using the alternative adjective of 'Fisher' rather than 'Grail' to describe the wounded King.

Some final points that will require elucidation: The place of the Crucifixion is called *Golgotha* meaning *skull*. This may indicate the topography of the site and a dark image of it being a place of execution, but it also brings into focus the head, as in Peredur's sight of the Grail, as well as associating with Brân the Blessed: The plot thickens.

Also, there is no lance or cup in Mark, these images seem to have been added into the Canon sometime later, with Mark's centurion becoming Longinus (meaning *long*) and using his spear (lance) to pierce Jesus' side; the cup then caught the blood and water that flowed from this wound (why water, I ask?). The imperative to include these items is unclear, except that they all refer back to deeper spiritual imagery, as evidenced in the *hallows* of the Tuatha.

The Grail legends have highlighted these symbols in the Grail procession; specifically, the cup as chalice that then conveniently fits the prior imagery in the expanded Crucifixion story. Maybe this was to link this event back to the Last Supper, or maybe it resonates more deeply with the various cauldrons in pre-Christian myth and legend, including and notably the Celtic, as a known symbol of sustenance and even transformation. The Lance is more associated with life:death at the Crucifixion and elsewhere and as a powerful symbol of wounding, suffering and healing.

All in all, this imagery draws a common pattern of betrayal (and/or vengeance), wounding (trauma) and suffering, healing (or resurrection).

Odin's Self-Sacrifice

This section has a twofold purpose. The first is to elaborate on the Lance in a more mythic and symbolic context, so that the above appreciation of it is not seen in relative isolation within the Grail legends. The second is to put the Passion into perspective, by looking outside our current cultural and religious framework and see that the core of the Passion – being the sacrificial death and resurrection of Jesus – is not unique and confined to Christianity.

Of course, this second point above is more widely appreciated in modern times, but I am proposing more than this. I have started to make some reference to this pattern in the Passion being more in our culture than we may hitherto have thought, with such accounts as the life and varied deaths of Merlin, specifically the triple death. I have also commented on the similarities between he and Woden (the British Odin). Even the Last Supper rings more of a shamanic ritual (maybe even involving hallucinogens in the wine). Here, I would like to step into a parallel culture and it's Pagan religious system, not only to give a comparative view of the Passion, but also to use it to further a healing process in our own culture between the Pagan and Christian worldviews.

Apart from seeing the significant role of the lance and the absence of a clear grail image, as well as the parallel nature of this myth with the Passion, I will be leaving the fuller exposition of this following account until later when it is linked with both Merlin and Woden (if, indeed, they differ). Instead, here I would like to emphasise the concept of *self-sacrifice* and highlight the perspective this gives to the Passion from a Pagan perspective, as well as pointing out that this is essentially *mythic*.

This slightly edited account is taken from Daniel McCoy's work on Norse Mythology, sourced online:

> *At the centre of the Norse cosmos stands the great tree Yggdrasil. Yggdrasil's upper branches cradle Asgard, the home and fortress of the Aesir gods and goddesses, of whom Odin is the chief.*
>
> *Yggdrasil grows out of the Well of Urd, a pool whose fathomless depths hold many of the most powerful forces and beings in the cosmos. Among these beings are the Norns, three sagacious maidens who create the fates of all beings. One of the foremost techniques they use to shape fate is carving runes into Yggdrasil's trunk. The*

symbols then carry these intentions throughout the tree, affecting everything in the Nine Worlds.

Odin watched the Norns from his seat in Asgard and envied their powers and their wisdom. And he bent his will toward the task of coming to know the runes.

Since the runes' native home is in the Well of Urd with the Norns, and since the runes do not reveal themselves to any but those who prove themselves worthy of such fearful insights and abilities, Odin hung himself from a branch of Yggdrasil, pierced himself with his spear, and peered downward into the shadowy waters below. He forbade any of the other gods to grant him the slightest aid, not even a sip of water. And he stared downward, and stared downward, and called to the runes.

He survived in this state, teetering on the precipice that separates the living from the dead, for no less than nine days and nights. At the end of the ninth night, he at last perceived shapes in the depths: the runes! They had accepted his sacrifice and shown themselves to him, revealing to him not only their forms, but also the secrets that lie within them. Having fixed this knowledge in his formidable memory, Odin ended his ordeal with a scream of exultation. Having been initiated into the mysteries of the runes, Odin recounted:

> *Then I was fertilized and became wise;*
> *I truly grew and thrived.*
> *From a word to a word I was led to a word,*
> *From a work to a work I was led to a work.*

Equipped with the knowledge of how to wield the runes, he became one of the mightiest and most accomplished beings in the cosmos. He learned chants that enabled him to heal emotional and bodily wounds, to bind his enemies and render their weapons worthless, to free himself from constraints, to put out fires, to expose and banish practitioners of malevolent magic, to protect his friends in battle, to wake the dead, to win and keep a lover, and to perform many other feats like these.

Our source for the above tale is the Hávamál, *an Old Norse poem. In the first of the two verses that describe Odin's shamanic initiatory ordeal itself (written from Odin's perspective), the god says that he was "given to Odin, myself to myself." The Old Norse phrase that translates to English as "given to Odin" is* gefinn Óðni, *a phrase that occurs many times throughout the Eddas and sagas in the context of human sacrifices to Odin. And, in fact, the form these sacrifices take mirrors Odin's ordeal in the* Hávamál; *the victim, invariably of noble birth, was stabbed, hung, or, more commonly, both at the same time.*

Odin's ordeal is therefore a sacrifice of himself to himself, and is the ultimate Odinnic sacrifice — for who could be a nobler offering to the god than the god himself?

I add the following, because it is often conflated with the above, and brings in the important feature of another of Odin's sacrifices, that of his eye:

On another occasion, he ventured to Mimir's Well – which is surely none other than the Well of Urd – amongst the roots of the world-tree Yggdrasil. There dwelt Mimir, a shadowy being whose knowledge of all things was practically unparalleled among the inhabitants of the cosmos. He achieved this status largely by taking his water from the well, whose waters impart this cosmic knowledge.

When Odin arrived, he asked Mimir for a drink from the water. The well's guardian, knowing the value of such a draught, refused unless the seeker offered an eye in return. Odin – whether straightaway or after anguished deliberation, we can only wonder – gouged out one of his eyes and dropped it into the well. Having made the necessary sacrifice, Mimir dipped his horn into the well and offered the now-one-eyed god a drink.

The latter piece adds *sacrifice* to the betrayal, wounding and healing complex, which is now expanding. But more to the – and my – point, is that Odin's myth takes the experience to one of *self-sacrifice*. This is not how we currently refer to the Crucifixion, instead it is laden with guilt, blame and judgement. Were we to see it in the context of a sacrifice in an initiatory and transformative life journey, it could then be a template for our own journeys, rather than seeing that in the hands of another, specifically Jesus, but maybe more directly the Christian God.

The ash tree that is Yggdrasil brings in the shamanic dimension to the myth. Yggdrasil is 'Odin's horse', a euphemism for the gallows, so an analogue to the Crucifixion cross. On this Odin hangs and then spears himself, instead of this being inflicted by others. The imagery in the myth, and as it resonates in the Crucifixion, is distinctly shamanic. The cross-referral to the triple death is also notable. The shamanic worldview can, in my opinion, provide a deep and unifying framework for all that I am discussing here. I will return to this in more detail and will also have more to say about the runes.

The Grail

The Physical Grail

The Grail as a physical entity may exist in the material world. But this would only be as a physical cup-like object that is imbued with magical power; maybe with the use of words in poetic or similar form when it becomes a charmed object. It's physical origin is hardly likely to be divine.

In this view, I am taking the world as a kind of reflection or mirror, a projection of spirit in physical space. Yet we are physically also such a reflection, as when we are dead. But alive we are more than this, because we can also conceive of this; it is as if our minds – or maybe our souls – are aware of this reflection in the moment, in time. When we lose this awareness, as for example in madness, we operate simply as selves in the world; in a weird manner, this way of being is as the walking dead.

What makes this step from self-in-the-world (not the Jungian *self*) to the soul and away from our mechanical, habitual, rational and cognitive way of being? I am suggesting it is when we step outside of space into a momentary time that such techniques as ritual and meditation facilitate. Here we are simply being, watching the world on one hand, and listening to spirit flow through and into us on the other. We are in a liminal and soulful state. We have moved from our heads to our heart. In this way, the physical heart can be seen as at least a metaphor for the Grail *within* us.

This is not to deny our mind and brain; they are an analogue of feeling and the heart. But as we reduce and understand our heart only in its mechanical function, we do the same to the brain and restrict its capacity to be a receiver of spirit that is channelled through the heart, to my more metaphoric way of understanding. This process I see as the mind moving to true intelligence and hence intellect, and the potential for either a mystical or a magical way of being.

So, there are no physical Grails in the world. Or, if there are, maybe the magical power that was vested in them has dissipated, withdrawn, and it is our responsibility to empower such potentially charmed objects again. After all, isn't that what the priest is doing with the chalice in Eucharist? Rather like Arthur and Merlin, it is time to drop the physical and historical search for the Grail. If we do want to find it, maybe we should begin with discovering our own hearts…

Images of the Grail

Robert de Boron in *Joseph of Arimathea* located the source of the Grail. He, and others, have identified this with the cup used in the Last Supper; although Mark's Gospel only refers to it as "he took the cup…", there is no more than that. And, as already stated, there is no mention of a lance in the Crucifixion; the centurion is only mentioned after Jesus dies, with the comment: "Truly this man was the Son of God". In fact, the whole account is a very simple factual one and quite bland. What is of interest to me is that there is no prior account of this cup-Grail or its origins.

Earlier, I described four ways in which the Grail can be seen: The cup of the Last Supper; the container that catches Jesus' blood from the lance-inflicted wound; the actual Messianic bloodline; or as something precious. At this point, the first two are now seen as relative, if consideration to Mark and subsequently the intention of medieval poets such as Robert de Boron are considered. Whether the familial connections in the medieval poets accounts of the Grail indicate a physical or symbolic bloodline is unclear. It is favoured by some modern investigators, but I believe this to be more psychologically and symbolically true, rather than physically or literally so. Such traits do follow bloodlines; we appreciate this in genetics in modernity, although there is a tendency to reduce these to a scientific framework only.

Certain traits are acknowledged to follow familial lines in other cultures, as in the capacity to be a shaman or healer; neither of which is unrelated to this point, I would add. Regal lineage uses this view to its advantage (or sometimes disadvantage), which is a position adopted by those who see the Grail as in the physical bloodline. I would argue this misses the point: The bloodline is a metaphor for traits passed down genetically, indicating the symbolic value of blood that is principally employed in this account as a healing agent, via sacrifice.

Seeing the Grail as something *precious* to my mind is closer to the truth, because it is directing attention to value, and not the physical object per se (although the two can, of course, be related). Wolfram describes it as a stone, here referencing alchemy or the *hallows*, to which we will come in more detail. But he goes no further, because it is the value that is important. Rather like bloodline, beyond a certain point following the line of the physical object is not helpful. But rather like bloodline, if considered symbolically, and where appropriate metaphorically, then a deeper appreciation may be revealed… but is this the Grail?

What I have found remarkable in my explorations is that the

Lance is not given sufficient emphasis. At times it approaches parity with the chalice image of the Grail, but not necessarily to supersede it. Yet in my perusal of the field, I find the Grail to relate more to sustenance with its platter and apparently endless food association, whereas the Lance is directly associated with wounding and healing, which I am increasingly seeing the core complex around which these images seem to satellite.

In addition, and as demonstrated in the Eucharist, the Grail is the container for blood, whereas it is the Lance with its dripping blood that both wounds and heals… as if the two functions can be separated. In a patriarchal system, I ask myself why this should be the case; unless it is an otherwise unconscious acknowledgement of the Celtic and feminine heritage that de Boron and others desired to Christianise. I suspect there are other threads here. The Lance also represents battle and vengeance, as discussed earlier. Maybe the healing needs to be done on these terms, by those who have wounded not only themselves, but the feminine. Is this where the Witch enters the picture, as Mary Magdalene, Morgana or even my Sacrificial Dream, and why she does?

When relativising the cup or chalice image as central to the Grail legends – as I have started to do here with the emphasis on the Lance – there are other images that need to be considered. *Excalibur*, of course, makes the sword central to the movie and even has a young Arthur referencing it as part of the dragon, in an early exchange with Merlin. The significant times Excalibur is used in the movie are: Merlin retrieving it from the lake via a feminine hand; Arthur drawing it from the stone; the knighting of Uriens; its braking in the duel with Lancelot with its casting into a lake and returning whole; Arthur stabbing into the earth between a sleeping Lancelot and Guinevere; the stabbing killing of Mordred in the final battle, and then Perceval finally returning it to the lake and the feminine hand that grasps it.

In the medieval accounts the sword is relatively peripheral to the Grail in the procession, although it is included at the beginning in Chrétien's poem. The mending of a broken sword is a strong image, where it represents an initiatory stage in a knight's spiritual development, with his ability to make it whole again. This is expanded by Boorman and Pallenberg into the unique scene of the fight between Lancelot and Arthur, where its breaking is a result of a moral violation; the mending occurs out of a vision in the lake into which it is cast, being presumably by the Lady of the Lake, to whom I shall return. This is mirrored when Guinevere returns the safely kept shroud-wrapped sword to Arthur before the final battle. It is thus a powerful symbol of wounding and healing... interestingly and ultimately in feminine hands, literally as well as symbolically.

The various accounts of the knights mending the sword is an interesting inquiry, but one that takes us too far afield with respect to this account. Apart from its significant relationship with the Lady of the Lake and as at least a reflection of wounding and healing, suffice it to say that the sword is associated with sovereignty; temporal as with Arthur and the Kingdom, or spiritual as with Perceval becoming the Grail King. In both cases this is related to the Land and at many places in the accounts; the image of the Waste Land is deeply reflected here, at times as much as the Grail itself, although they are deeply related themes.

Although removing the sword from the stone is quite a dramatic visual scene in *Excalibur*, it may be a relatively simple procedure that was undertaken in kingship ceremonies, something like a coronation. Yet, the movie does highlight an association not seen as clearly in the various poems, which is the relationship between the sword and (the) stone. Having said this, there is the prior substitution of the precious Stone for the Grail that Wolfram undertook, in contrast to the more secular function of it in king-making. Following this change is a deeper issue, that in pre-Christian culture and even extending to modernity (the Kaaba in Mecca, for example) this Stone is of symbolically divine origin, even as a metaphoric or literal meteorite from the 'heavens'. Stone circles, of course, abound in pre-Christian cultures.

Like the sword, such stones are associated with sovereignty (the British Coronation being effected on the Stone of Scone or Destiny), making them reflections of a complex and deeply symbolic image. Such extensive associations point to the symbolic depth and power of the image, and its representation in reality. It may be that the sword was not buried in the stone, although this may reflect an intense sexual, tantric or alchemical association, but simply laid on it as with an altar.

There is, however, another more magical and alchemical explanation of the sword-in-the-stone. The end of the Stone Ages are marked first by the Bronze and subsequently the Iron Age. This marks the age of metals and the rise of the mystical tradition of alchemy that sees working with them as the reflection of a psychospiritual process. The blacksmith has always been seen as a marginal and hence often a shamanic figure with mythic and magical overtones. It is he who would take the stone and from it produce the iron that by tempering into steel became the sword. The sword from the stone...

The Grail Procession

The now-capitalised Procession can be relatively simple, as in Chrétien, or more complex, as in Wolfram which I shall come to. Basically, it is a ritual as well as being ceremonial; although I had better qualify the distinction. A ceremony is something partaken in when someone or something is presented to an audience, as with a marriage, for example. Yet at the core of a ceremony can be embedded a ritual, as with the actual ritual performed by priest, bride and groom. The Mass with the Eucharist are similar.

The ritual process takes the participant from observer to active engagement; in effect, he, she or they enter into a differing or altered state of consciousness or trance-state of varying depth. In this metaphoric place, relatively out-of-time, the participant(s) can then enter into the depth of meaning and purpose of the ritual. Although embedded in ceremony in the above examples, a ritual can exist on its own. Initiation and Rites of Passage are examples.

There is also a progressive depth of involvement in the *symbolic* process in ritual and ceremony; a word I have used frequently and may also need to explain a little. I would start by saying that in our present era we live in a metaphoric flatland, where depth and subtlety have become ruled by an overly rational, cognitive and mechanical worldview; science has become *scientism* and the mystical aspect our of being reduced to doctrinaire religion. In effect, our three-dimensional world has become two, where such terms as myth and magic have, somewhat paradoxically, come to mean their opposites. We are bereft; indeed, we may be living in the Waste Land. As climate change, the Land grieves and we live in fear of creations smallest organisms that seem to burrow in the very core of our being, our genetic selves.

Symbolism has become sign, or the known; yet another inversion. But symbolism is not a sign, and if it is, it is simply the known end of a spectrum that flows to and from the unknown. While symbols may be appreciated indirectly by their signs and hinted at through analogy and metaphor, they are ultimately unknowable and mysterious. We feel their effects rather than think them. They radiate through the soul and are felt in the heart and enrich the mind; they touch our emotional beings and ultimately are agents of healing, in that healing means to make whole and unite our psychic divisions. Ultimately, a symbol will *move* us, otherwise we are not appreciating it. When so moved, the soul is awoken from its sleep and life propels us forward guided by the power of the symbol, that in and of itself, is the numinous language of the *Divine*.

What enlivens symbolism – think of the Charm here – is ritual. This is what makes true creativity ultimately spiritual, because the artist ritualises the creative process. In contrast to formal religion where symbolism becomes doctrinaire, rote and two-dimensional, creativity moves, changes and renews. It has deep roots in the feminine, water and fluidity. Symbols emerge in the artist's hand, move and morph, die and revive, wound and heal; deeply alchemical, the opposites are brought into proximity, gender union, rebirth... Yet ritual can contain structure, providing a physical and psychic space to enter into, a setting, somewhere to divest oneself of daily concerns, to move into a soulful space beyond time and hear the inspiration of spirit, and cooperate with it.

When the Procession is considered, I have found it important to see it as visionary and hence with a symbolic gaze, which the above remarks preface. The actual facts and details of it are interesting, but maybe not as relevant as where they are pointing in terms of symbolic intent. Rather like a dream the Procession is best understood in this light, because I am sure each individual poet has adorned it with their own views and even prejudices.

In Chrétien (as earlier):

> *A squire enters carrying a sword with engraved blade, and announces that the lord's niece has sent it to him – the lord gives the sword to Perceval. Another squire enters carrying a white lance on whose tip blood oozed and flowed down onto the squire's hand. A maiden brings in a grail held in both hands (a serving dish),*

and the room becomes brightly illuminated. Another brings in a silver carving platter. The grail is made of gold and set with precious stones – it and the platter are carried to another chamber.

What is notable to me is that there are complex of icons or symbols in Chrétien. The sword is somewhat peripheral and given to Perceval, in a manner that recalls Arthur and his sword, Excalibur. Perceval will become the Grail King. As Arthur is to become the temporal King, Perceval correspondingly is the spiritual one. What further strikes me is that the spear is prominent and associated with blood, not the cup or chalice. In fact, there is no direct reference to a cup, but rather a Grail that is a serving dish and provides food aplenty, Celtic-style.

In Wolfram:

Following the showing of the blood-covered spear, four sets of female characters enter the room: first, the ones carrying the chandeliers; then the ones with the ivory pedestals, torches, the tabletop made of precious gems and silver knives. Eighteen ladies are mentioned as performing this service, to which number another six become added. At the centre is the female keeper and guardian of the Grail. After the procession scene, the knights present are invited to the supper. One hundred tables are set up for the feast, each served by four knights. The Grail provides all the desired food.

As mentioned earlier, the Grail is something like a precious stone, in Wolfram, which still resonates with Chrétien's description of the Grail, though differs significantly from the head on the platter in Peredur. This ceremony is all set in a feminine realm, in contrast to the lance and sword; interestingly, the latter is brought in at the end and not prior to the Procession.

This generally leads me to the conclusion that the Grail, as the central symbol of the profession, is more than just a single icon and is artistically crafted to represent the creative and spiritual intent of each poet; certainly, this is also the case with the subsequent Christianisation of the story by various poets and commentators. I also see each representation to have deep, mythic and maybe historical roots as in the cauldron of plenty (Celtic), head (vengeance) and stone (alchemical). The Christian chalice should possibly be seen in a similar light.

But before I do this, I would like to render the Procession in a different manner as in a dream, where I am the dreamer. One reason to do this, is to place it into a format that more closely approximates the dream theme-work of this account. Yet there is a deeper reason than this indicated by modernity's relative minimisation of the Procession, whereas to me it is exactly this that lifts these works beyond the more mundane tales of knights and chivalry. This is because it is a ritual process, akin to, but also maybe superseding the Mass. Think this threatens the Church? Sure do.

First in a condensed account of Chrétien's Procession, written in the first person with myself as dreamer. The sources for the 'dream' are varied, but accord with the original:

> *I am talking with an older man of some wealth*
> *and status, who is reclining on a couch when a young*
> *man comes into the room with a sword hanging from*

his neck like a necklace. He hands it to the man, who part withdraws it from the scabbard and sees from an engraving where it has been made. It seems unbreakable, unless afflicted by something only known to its maker. The man gives me the sword.

I resume conversation with him when another young man brings in a shining lance and walks in front of a fire, as I notice others on and around the couch on which the older man is reclining. We all notice a drop of blood emerge from the tip of the lance and run down to the young man's hand.

Then two more young men come in carrying golden candelabras with lighted candles, followed by a beautiful well-dressed young lady carrying a golden serving bowl adorned with precious jewels in her hands that outshone the lance.

She is followed by a young woman holding a silver carving platter. The bowl and platter bearers pass by and out of my vision.

I am dumbfounded with what I am witnessing. The scene fades and I wake up astonished, but calm.

When I do this creative interpretation, I am both surprised and impressed that I use the word 'dumbfounded'. To me, this indicates something different to the failure of Perceval's asking of the question; it is neither guilt nor prior instruction, but awe. Because the scene is awesome in its numinosity, which is enough to strike any onlooker dumb, a feature noted elsewhere in other similar spiritual accounts. I suspect, rather like myself in the Original Dream, the experience is enough to simply witness; the questions come later, and I believe this is the case with Perceval and is the intent of the poet.

But there is no Grail as such; there is a magnificent serving bowl and a lesser but still significant carving platter, both related to food. This is distinctly Celtic, but resonates in many traditions. It provides an interesting backdrop to the Christian Host and, rather like the Host, indirectly seems to be for the old man, maybe to sustain him. Yet the sword is given to me, what am I meant to do with it? The lance is entrancing, but I cannot ascertain its significance from the dream account alone. They do resonate with dreams I have had before and have recounted here, however...

Although a somewhat simplistic interpretation, let me take a step back and look at the content. It is obvious now that this Procession is to an audience and not simply the man; it has wider and maybe general application. Whilst the sword and lance resonate with the hallows, the bowl and platter are less clearly associated with the chalice and stone, but they are also not entirely separate and may be alternative representations. I am drawn to the food aspect of the items, although there is no drink, maybe with the notable exception of the blood. Am I missing something?

Now to Wolfram's poem, similarly condensed from varied sources:

A young man dashes through an open door carrying a lance, that makes others watching this in the dream distressed, as we all witness blood that drips from the point down the shaft to the man's hand and runs into his sleeve.

I look around what I now see I am in a great hall seated on a couch next to a venerable man who is old, unwell and part reclining. The audience around us is comprised of elegant young women, dressed somewhat ritualistically with flowers coiffured in their long, blond hair.

I notice four of them have burning candlesticks, and the four others are carrying a shining deep-red precious stone shaped like a table-top, which is then set over trestles.

A number of other women seem to enter from around, undertaking performance acts that are vague to me and then walk away; there may be men dressed as knights beyond. Then follows a single radiantly regal woman, dressed in fine middle-eastern silks and upon a green silk she carries what I know is the Grail and sets it on the table.

It seems to me that apart from the radiance, there is nothing there. Then it takes a shape, sometimes as a precious green jewel emerging from a stone, and sometimes as a vessel that I can only vaguely determine. I am filled with humility and am in awe.

Then I am distracted as a young man brings in a sword in its sheath, its handle studded with rubies. It feels to have a rich history as the man part withdraws it and presents it to the old man; he declines and motions to give the sword to me.

As I gaze in awe at the sword, the scene beyond becomes vague and disappears. I look around and see that I am now alone in the woods beyond.

It is difficult to give full justice to Wolfram's Procession scene; it is rich and complex. Yet, when I ceased trying to make a literal interpretation in my imaginative dream I found it difficult when

I reach the point the Grail entered. I stopped, took some time out, and returned to it, determining to picture it as I saw it, yet relatively true to the description in the translated verses.

I suspect this was because I have embellished it and, although it appears comparative to my Original Dream and the jewel in the fountain, it is also true to the poem and spirit of the verse. The vessel image is mine, I admit, but the poet describes the Grail but no object. It remains unclear to me from the literature as to why commentators are so definite in seeing the image of the Grail as a stone in Wolfram; the common interpretation that it is a precious stone or jewel, probably green, and referred to as *lapis exillis* or the stone of the philosopher. I have represented these ambiguities with dreamlike changes.

Yet the image is compatible with my Original Dream in many obvious ways, and at a time that I had no knowledge of this poem, let alone the content. This is so significant to me that I will be exploring my life in this context and research into the future.

It is interesting that I have placed myself in Parzival's place; it was natural to do this. The sword is presented similarly to Chrétien's poem, though at the end rather than the beginning of the Procession. Passing it to me is as if I am assuming the old man's position as a rite of succession. In contrast the scene with the lance is doleful, and I suspect that the sword is a responsibility to deal with the events that the lance has unleashed.

Between these scenes are the various ones with women and one in particular, whom Wolfram identifies as the Queen of the Grail; am I it's King now? And what does that mean? Is this literal or metaphoric, temporal or spiritual? My feeling is that the Grail heals and transforms whatever is associated with the lance and places the responsibility of enactment on the new sword-bearer. It is this that I failed to do in the Original Dream, which in Wolfram is asking the King what ails him? When Parzival does eventually ask this of the King, he is miraculously healed without a response. So maybe it is not a question of answers to problems, but asking the right questions…

I interpret this now as the sickness of the world around me, a modern Waste Land. The blatant failure of medicine to deal with sickness, as identified to me in the recent pandemic; Climate Change that is the subject of rhetoric and little action; the rise of autocracies to world dominance and the shading of fledgling democracy; the failure of the Church and established religion to provide succour… these all come to mind.

But what am I to do? As it seems I can no longer shirk responsibility; if I do, the Grail will pass away and the Waste Land continue. Of course, I do not see myself as the saviour, but representative of every man. So maybe my choice is in the company of others making this core realisation and that is what the remainder of my life is about, connecting with them, asking the right questions and enacting my truth.

Theme Reflection

A long pause ensued at this point in my inquiry. I felt that I was almost in over my head with themes and that my intent was becoming obscured. I determined it was time to take a deep breath and reflect on all these themes that seemed to be mounting up to the point of confusion.

The most surprising insight came very recently. Yesterday, I was at an inlet where the river forged a path into the Great Southern Ocean. I gazed at the horizon where the headland met the skyline, as did a nearby island, and it seemed to me that all along the horizon other mountainous hilltops emerged in the light haze. Of course, I knew this was an optical illusion based on my shifting gaze from landscape to sea and horizon, but it was still magical, as if a great continent sat just beyond my clear gaze.

There are many parallels to what I am writing. The mist itself is a consistent theme and the vision of a continent may be that of the distant Antarctica across the ocean... or even the island of my Original Dream. Or, then again, it could be Avalon, the mystical land of Faery. I let my imagination run, entranced by the vision and my love of this place. I also realised I had *come home* in the sense that, rather like the Welsh *hiraeth*, this deeply emotional connection to this place sang to me.

Then I recalled that I had now returned for the second time. I had first come here thirty years before, similarly entranced and enchanted by the place. But the demands of parenthood, career and marriage, as well as a serious but redeemable illness, led me back to the capital city and a future that was to see all of these calls to duty fail… or apparently so. I had arrived at the Grail Castle it appeared, seemingly too soon. I had not asked the questions demanded of me; indeed, at that time I didn't even know they existed. Now I was back like Perceval – or Parzival, as I generally refer to him henceforth – to ask the question; maybe only of myself, but ask it I must.

My intent in this inquiry is not to provide academic information about the subject matter I am travelling through, or insights of an intellectual, scholarly or even psychological nature. It is to link these great texts of a bygone era or eras into the present – my present – and see them as maps of a fateful nature now that my soul has awoken to the task at hand. But, more than this, such material can be the same for us all. In the West, we walk an individualistic path that we somehow have to reconcile in a psychospiritual manner. Once the demands of duty and obligation are completed – or never undertaken – this is the true demand that supersedes all others. Many a mystic and artist knows this and rejects such a dutiful path from the onset; maybe I am just a later bloomer, or indicating that such a path is there for us all.

This is the core truth I wish to convey: It is my intention. As I pass now to the various other themes I have touched upon or that are yet to emerge, I realise that I have flirted with many; some rejected, and others seductive. The last to so enchant me has been Wolfram's work, and hence the reason I now use the name Parzival in preference to Perceval. But as I have moved more deeply into the accounts of the Grail Procession, it is time to bring some of the other themes into context and, by virtue of their omission, to reject others.

Dreams are central. Not only as the psychospiritual backbone to my journey, but also because they reveal images and symbols that connect to the other themes that I am entertaining and exploring.

I had thought there were no more to recount, then during this reflective phase I had the following dream:

> *I am investigating a man's death with a large arrow-like spear that may be self-inflicted, although the couple of onlookers indicate that the arrow in its mechanism — something like a large crossbow — is too big to be able to do this. There are two such arrows arranged across each other, like great pins or crowbars. I show that a particular arm manoeuvre would get the hand to the trigger to be able to fire it when turned back on himself.*
>
> *(Sacrificial Dream: Addendum 2022)*

Whilst I mention the dream now, I will probably refer to it when the Sacrificial Dream is further explored, because it obviously relates with the common imagery. I have been investigating the man's death, or intend to do so further, and maybe am being instructed to by the dream. Death has been close to me in this intervening period, as I have reflected on and grieved more on the passing of a couple of close friends in the last few years, as well as the loss of both my parents and the demise of my long-term marriage in this same period.

However, the difference between this Addendum and the Sacrificial Dream is that this wounding and death is by a self-inflicted wound, rather than being administered by another. What compounds this further is that the act that does this is something that reflects a current injury I have sustained to my shoulder in a self-inflicted manner. In the dream, this manoeuvre is possible, but was I to try it in reality, it would produce pain and retraumatise the injury; in effect, I cannot do it. The other reflection on death has been my own. After a viral affliction, maybe coronavirus, a couple of months before, I started to sustain a cough and irregular heartbeat. Whilst this has settled with a shamanic approach, it has – once again – brought me in touch with my own mortality and, on this occasion, how much of our own death is self-inflicted.

What alerted me to the similarity of this with the Sacrificial Dream was: *There are two such arrows arranged across each other, like great pins or crowbars.* Not only is the pin similar, but now there are two across each other; a thinly disguised reference the cross of the Crucifixion, maybe, reinforced by the tool being a *cross*-bow. Somewhat tangentially, does the *crow*-bar association refer to Odin's shamanic association with that bird, I wonder? All this I will take into account when I return to the Sacrificial Dream; it is as if I need further psychic information when I do this…

And this is where one of those rabbit holes opens up. It would be easy – for me particularly with my professional past – to wander into dream territory with information, insights and even theories. Many have done this and if I were to do this, it would not be here. It is sufficient to me not only that we all dream, but that they flow in and through as a subterranean stream, bringing the patterns of our life from the perspective of soul into our awareness. Not only are they guides, they also reveal to us what our own psychic blueprint looks like.

What I am realising is that we already have a satisfactory term for the worldly self, which in its various representations the psychologically-oriented have confused with the territory that soul previously occupied. I suspect that this is partly because, and maybe a consequence of the era presently being examined: The Church has appropriated the soul, disconnected it from the body and emotions, and allied it with the transpersonal realm of spirit and the religious one of the monotheistic God. Psychology generally seems to have eschewed soul as a utilisable term, appropriating the Greek *Psyche* instead.

What has intrigued me in this inquiry is that it is obvious that in this very short period of history – some fifty years around the turn of the 13thC – there is a rich corpus of work from the pens of the various bards, troubadours and minnesingers. Further, that these works threatened the Church immensely and led to repercussions starting with the Inquisition, which has not ended, even in the present. What was it so threatened the religious establishment?

In a practical sense, one aspect is writing. Whilst previously under the aegis of the Church, in this period the various lyric poets – and using different tongues – came under the authority of other than the Church, with the patronage of nobles. Issues such as love, the meaning of wounding and healing, and the personal realisation of spiritual enlightenment without the agency of religion was, and remains, a threat to the core. The idea that the individual could obtain such spiritual realisation without the agency of the Christian path through Jesus led to repercussions in that era that, to my way of seeing it, simply endorsed the Gnostic view that the God of the establishment is a phoney, a copy, a pseudo-God.

The esoteric came to light and briefly eclipsed the establishment, the exoteric. But the latter dealt with this, not only by suppression and hence psychological repression, but also in a manner in which it is now well-versed; that is, appropriation. The body of work that was revealed in Chrétian started the ball rolling with Perceval and his connection to Pagan and Celtic sources. But Wolfram was to take this further with a Parzival that also dealt with the spirituality of the East beyond Christianity and brought in the tradition of alchemy as a tool.

The Church, particularly the Cistercians and the pen of Robert de Boron, began this appropriation by Christianising the narrative and connecting the Grail, as exclusively cup or chalice, to the events of the Passion. The deed was done. The soul is taken from immediate access and taken to its logical extreme in the form of the pure, ideal and virginal Galahad. At the close of the era, even Malory put the Grail achievement in his hands. Interestingly, *Excalibur*, which supposedly is based on Malory's *Morte d'Arthur*, assigns the Grail achievement to the pre-Christian Perceval. The film also attempts to deal with other themes, such as love and wounding:healing (and with it the place of the sword and lance) with themes that even resonate with the fabled Tristan and Iseult, taking us back – again – to Pagan sources.

Whilst psychology has tried to rescue the soul from obscurity, this has been largely done in a cognitive manner, and hence one acceptable to the institutional establishment. There are exceptions – most notably Jung – although even he used the term *self*, which I believe is a concept that more accurately approximates the traditional concept of the *soul* at the personal level. The concept of the *self* is Jung's attempt to include his idea of the Collective Unconscious into its remit. His further rediscovered concept of *Individuation* provides a pathway into the esoteric, but also and maybe more importantly, recognises that the West has yet to come to terms with the status of the individual and their pathway to the divine.

In a nutshell, this is my life's journey, although I fully recognise I am not alone. In an era where the Church is finally losing its grip, the possibility of re-establishing our earthly connection to the soul and see it as the vehicle to the divine, beyond its present reductionistic position in psychology, may finally have arrived. The seeds cast eight hundred years ago may now be flowering.

Of course, I am using some recognised approaches, such as alchemy, to support this thesis. But I am also drawing on some others, such as shamanism and magic, to further enhance it. Whilst Wolfram went to the East, I will be heading North. And I will also be making a belated return to Merlin.

It might appear that in the Christian debate, I am taking the Pagan corner and rejecting the religion of my birth. I am not. What I am doing is seeing the latter *relatively*, and not the only tradition that claims a pathway to the divine. But with my non-conformist and individualistic tendency, it is hard to accept the duty-ridden story based on an interpretation of events two millennia past in a literal and factual manner only.

Instead, I see that the eruption of the Grail material eight hundred years ago represented a spiritual urge to re-establish an inner and esoteric connection to the divine in the European West. Of course, the poems and other stories can be relatively ridiculed in a factual and historical manner; but they are not exoteric, they are mythic, creative and esoteric. Ironically, the brutal suppression of this material in the ensuing centuries is not unlike what happened to Christianity itself in the early centuries of the Common Era.

When seen in this manner, the actual story of Jesus takes on a more mythic hue, one that shows the emergence of the spiritual through the fabric of a degenerate tradition that has lost touch with the esoteric. With this common resonance with the period I am examining, even that of Merlin/Woden and Odin only some five hundred years later, I believe it is totally valid to see the Christian story as one amongst many. Rather like the Arthurian and Grail legends, Christianity has been pruned into an inconsistent story around a man from the Middle East. Though he was charismatic, a healer, maybe politically motivated and a mystic, there is little doubt. Except that he, like Parzival and Merlin, may be a condensation of many historical figures around a mythic and archetypal core. And, rather like the more Pagan Grail threads, the vast corpus of Gnostic material was itself suppressed, once formal Christianity got the upper hand.

Parzival indicates a greater vision, by pointing to the East beyond Palestine and finding common ground there with its traditions and spirituality; there are even threads of Buddhism in it, as well as most certainly alchemy. Wolfram's vision embraces a worldview where East and West are connected, even united. He points to the Indo-European undercurrents of all the traditions examined here, including the Celtic, Nordic and Christian, with its mythic, alchemical and spiritual threads. It is a deep and grand vision and one I am personally drawn to.

There are some peripheral features that indicate this, beyond the adoption of the Grail motif. The crown of thorns relates eastwards to Buddhism, as observers like the great mythographer Joseph Campbell has pointed out. The title 'King of the Jews' seems a little anomalous until we consider the Grail King. The cross at Calvary (the place of the skull; remember Peredur?) is not unlike the tree on which Odin was hung with his self-inflicted wounds; for both, it is a reference to the Tree of Life, on which we are all suspended. The terms 'Son of Man' and 'Son of God' point to our dual identity as physical beings leading a time-bound life between birth and death, and a transcendent one: We are all both. Maybe the obscure naked figure in the Garden of Gethsemane and in the tomb of Jesus is a reference to this duality. And what about all the women in the events of the Passion, at a time when the patriarchy reigned supreme? I am just putting the Christian story into a more appropriate context and one I can live with. In effect, this is that the myth of the Passion is a map that defines the path that all on the path of Individuation must face.

At this juncture, I feel to set out the themes that I have covered to a varied extent already, but need to revisit in a more cohesive manner as the finishing line to this inquiry starts to beckon, although this cohesion will not necessarily be in the condensed and linear order that immediately follows. By now, it must be apparent that these themes need to be examined in a fluid rather than a fixed manner, as a process rather than a structure. In fact, it is such a fixed, structured and reductive approach that has led to much being missed.

Through a revisitation of Odin's self-sacrifice and how this pertains to both Merlin and my Sacrificial Dream, I propose to look in some detail at the Northumbrian runes of the extension to the Anglo-Saxon Futhorc for a window into the proto-Grail material that emerged in northern Europe in the first millennium. This will lead into a discussion of alchemy and its relevance, leading up to Wolfram's Parzival and beyond. Merlin will then emerge from his Esplumoir and back into the Grail corpus that parallels this discussion and flows into it more significantly. I will examine the relationship between Merlin, the Grail King and Parzival in a more detailed manner, relating them all back to the male figures of my dreams. From the Grail Procession and even the accounts in other stories, such as the Resurrection, the feminine requires honouring and balancing with the masculine figures to date, so that the thorny issues of sex and power can be looked at further.

From this alchemical, Jungian and even Tantric perspective, I would like to ask questions about wounding, healing and love. But these elements take me back to the archetypal framework of shamanism that I believe underpins much of this account; not only because of my own professional story, but also because it demands to be reinstated in this period of history.

Finally, I intend to ask how all this relates to the present era and its demands. I believe we are going through a transitional stage that the account to date foreshadows at various times in our history. However, one of my main theses is that this are not simply historical, they are also mythic; they are not only in the past, but also deep in the present. Hence my reference to people like Jung and Campbell.

These patterns and the truths they hold have much to inform us. It is a task I have to complete in my own journey and may also be relevant to anyone reading this account.

Healing and the Grail

I am not sure whether the title of this section exactly embraces the themes immediately above, which I intend to explore now in more detail, but it will suffice. Healing has been more than my trade; it is my vocation. Incompatible with modern western medicine, I have sought its roots via Jung and the various traditions I encountered there, which litter this account. In so doing, I have been drawn to a deeper perspective of my destiny or *wyrd* and the consequence is this work, the final one in my memoir series. This section will be the framework for a temporal journey into the present and a vision of the future; it is a path with and of my soul.

Sacrificial Dream Reprise

I related this dream earlier in the previous section. I had thought I had done with it, but the recent emergence of a dream with similar imagery made me realise that it still had some secrets to reveal. Not mentioned at the time I recounted this Addendum dream to the Sacrificial one was that it seemed to take place in the field beyond where I had seen Merlin in my childhood memory. It is also where I received my adolescent sex education on a walk with my mother. Based on consequences such as pregnancy and infectious disease, it was hardly a warm and loving introduction; as if I needed one by that time anyway, my prior learning gave me a sense of perspective.

I mention these associations now, because they are two areas I want to cover further and they also embellish the Addendum dream:

> *I am investigating a man's death with a large arrow-like spear that may be self-inflicted, although the couple of onlookers indicate that the arrow in its mechanism — something like a large crossbow — is too big to be able to do this. There are two such arrows arranged across each other, like great pins or crowbars. I show that a particular arm manoeuvre would get the hand to the trigger to be able to fire it when turned on the shooter.*

I mentioned earlier the shoulder injury that is reflected in the dream, although in a 'healed' capacity. In fact, I have now injured both and this reminds me of the man in the Sacrificial Dream: Not only that, it also identifies me with him. I had seen that the original man becomes the sacrificial one even unto death, it would seem to be saying in this Addendum, if there were any doubt prior to this. I am also increasingly identifying with him here, although in reality my shoulder concerns would directly place me in this sacrificial position.

Is this a warning to me? Physically, maybe yes, as death has been on my horizon for quite some time, in a metaphoric and symbolic sense. I am also sensing some urgency, and that this Addendum is suggesting I attend to these issues. The main feature, however, is that the wound is now self-inflicted. In a subtle sense, I had come to this conclusion about the Crucifixion; that it is an act of self-sacrifice in service of a spiritual transformation, that in a metaphoric sense it is an illustration to me, and to us all, of what we may have to go through.

In this context, I am not looking at the dream for

psychological content to deal with concerns in my daily life, although the reference to death should alert me to the literal interpretation in everyday reality. It is more as material to link my personal journey with transpersonal elements – creative (including this work), mythic, archetypal, spiritual – and to appreciate these with a metaphoric and symbolic gaze. And, in terms of tradition and background, the Sacrificial Dream and it's Addendum relate more to the story about Odin's self-sacrifice elucidated earlier, rather than to the Christian story, although it parallels this in an archetypal sense. This will ultimately lead me back to Merlin via Woden, but prior to this I want to explore the significance of the runes to this account.

Runes, Alchemy and The Grail

In a rather direct manner, I am now shifting my gaze from Odin (Old Norse) to Woden (Anglo-Saxon and hence Old English) as they are relatively synonymous; sufficiently so for my purpose in this account, anyway.

All manner of possibilities would open up were I to stay in the Norse arena with its rich mythology, contrasting to the somewhat fragmented one in Britain influenced as it was by various cultural streams, including the less integrative and ultimately more suppressive Christian one. But this is my story, so it is not only Woden I am drawn to with his parallels and even continuity to Merlin, but the runes of the first millennium in Britain that took a differing path that the standard Germanic (Norse) rune row called the Futhark. It is one inclusive of Christian influence, mainly in its Celtic form and specifically in Northumbria away from Rome's watchful eye – for a while, at least.

Known as the Futhorc, the Anglo-Saxon (AS) runes were extended beyond the twenty-four of the Germanic Elder Futhark, initially to twenty-eight or nine (or thereabouts) to accommodate the British influence around trees, the environment generally, and possibly Ogham – a form of graphic communication reckoned to be Celtic. Common to both Ogham and the AS runes is its graphic and symbolic level of communication, although the runes seemingly superseded Ogham, with the Scandinavian influence of the first millennium. Then followed an extension from the twenty-nine or so, to thirty-three or four; this is known as the Northumbrian extension. For the purposes of this account and my inquiry, I am looking at runes twenty-eight to thirty-three, although there is inevitably some variation in ordering and what each rune represents.

The indented comments that follow are drawn directly from my book on the Futhorc, called *Spellbinding*, with some editing and minor modifications for this work. Here are the relevant runes of the extension in succession:

> Rune twenty-eight called *Ior* – ᛡ – is a transitional one in the extension and could be left out of this present discussion, except that it refers to a serpent and, therefore analogously, to the dragon. This alternative is provided in the first line of the Charm of Making within this account. I have left it in because in the magical context, the serpent is a strong sexual image that recalls the kundalini energy coiled at the base of the spine, evoked and awakened by ritual sexual activity; it is a, or the, fundamental energetic power in the human psycho-physical organism. There is a sense with Ior of balance and equality, with the gender-ambiguous nature of the serpent. Yet the serpent, or snake as

kundalini, is the primal force of our spiritual evolution where the male and female elements are also in balance. This may be the core feature of Ior, balance in the primal sense, as reinforced by its home in the waters of the maternal womb.

Rune twenty-nine *Ear* – ᛠ – like *Ior* and the runes preceding it in the extension, has what is known as the Old English rune poem associated with it; poetry that is relatively Christianised. The poem for this rune is sombre, taking the literal meaning of *Ear*, as earth and soil, into death and disintegration. But in the Pagan mentality, this gloominess is not necessarily the case: Death can be seen as a transition, either as a metempsychosis or to a more glorious existence, as exemplified in the image of the Norse Valhalla. Ear is the death that marks the ritual dismemberment and burning at the beginning of the alchemical process that is also reflected in shamanism.

Ear marks the end of the rune poem and most extant versions of the Futhorc. However, there are four further runes, derived from what is known as the Northumbrian rune row and preserved now only in manuscript form, that are particularly worth considering in this account. Without them Ear would be leaving the Christian story at the Crucifixion and not considering the Resurrection. Modernity sometimes makes a similar mistake, and here the more mystical inclination of Northumbria is significant.

Cweorth – ᛢ – rune thirty, is the ritual fire of

change and transformation. Cweorth indicates a process of change or transition that succeeds Ear. It is clearly delineated in the alchemical process and indicates a difficult, life-threatening, but also a life-changing transition that demands support rather than protection from these forces. It is a powerful image that, to my mind, reinforces much of the pathways of spiritual evolution that are symbolised in the Passion, and hence reinforcing the progressive Christian influence in these latter runes from a more mystical and esoteric, rather than an exoteric perspective.

But this is Christian influence now devoid of the rune poem for any assistance in interpretation, and is in contrast to the verse in Ear. With this relative disadvantage of a corresponding poem, maybe the imperative is to return to the image, name and symbol, and draw the sort of conclusions being elucidated here without this level of religious influence. Maybe we are getting back to the alchemical and mystical source that underlies the religious message... maybe beyond death to not only resurrection, but also a pathway to spiritual realisation?

Rune thirty-one, *Calc* – ᛣ – designates a cup, or chalice, maybe inverted. In all these connections and associations death is not a final act, but a transformation. In the Teutonic tradition, the drinking horn would serve a social and religious function as well, and parallels much of the Christian imagery; here are points of merging and connection that indicate a creative flowing together of these changing times, rather than seeing them as fundamentally adversarial as becomes the case. There is also the sense that this is of a higher order of transition or spiritual evolution; there is also something in the name. Calcination is a stage – the first – in alchemy. It is the stage when the base material is placed in a container, which is then closed, and then fire applied to it to effect change.

There is an alternative form of Calc, sometimes referred to as a *Double Calc* or *KK* – ᛤ – which is an embellished combination of Calc and an earlier rune of the Futhorc, the thirteenth *Eolh* – ᛉ – that is Calc inverted or righted. I have put KK here next to Calc, although it is by no means certain that is its place; maybe it should be separate, or even put to the end of the sequence because of the similarity to rune thirty-three, *Gar*. I will leave the question of place open, but point out that it does satisfy many of the qualities described in Calc. Calc is a deep image and indicates that the alchemical transformative process is proceeding in a spiritual manner. As a chalice, or even the Grail, transubstantiation is both a physical and a spiritual process: Born of sacrifice, it is entering into the Kingdom; or, in Pagan terminology, Valhalla.

Continuing the alchemical theme is the concept of the *stone of the philosopher* with *Stan* – ᛥ – rune thirty-two. This is the base material – the prima materia – and is the beginning of the alchemical work that ultimately results in the so-called *philosopher's stone*. This somewhat confusing and paradoxical terminology is common in alchemy and reinforces its reputation as being somewhat obfuscatory. This resultant philosopher's stone is believed to catalyse the transformation of base metals into gold, as well as being the *elixir of life*.

This latter Elixir association provides a connection of Stan with Calc and the Holy Grail, as well as the ultimate outcome and completion of the alchemical process. What is intriguing is that the stone is central to the art of alchemy and its association with the transformation images and myths of Christianity and the Grail Legends. Why is this? Alchemy would seem to be a very metallic art with the various materials used, and it's associations are with the planets and astrology. Yet the whole process is centred around the philosopher's stone with its philosophical and spiritual connotations.

Mythologically the thirty-third *spear* rune – ᚸ – is that of Woden and is representative of Yggdrasill, the world-tree. It is also the spear which marks part of Woden's self-sacrifice to obtain Galdor, the magical wisdom of the word contained in the runes. This, as well as the image itself, tends to mark Gar apart from the other runes that precede it, although it also remains symbolically connected. Gar, like its sibling Double Calc, is a contained image that is quite mandalic, and could also represent the unified *self* in the Jungian psychological sense. It contains within itself much of the imagery of the runes that precede it, and orders them into a unified whole.

What might be appreciated from this is the obvious Christian influence that has permeated the runes through Northumbria. Historically this is perhaps no surprise, and the Christian influence should definitely be seen as Celtic-inclined, mystical and esoteric, hence the profound association with alchemical imagery. This is reinforced by the Grail references I have drawn upon here. But, more than this, I believe that the continuity of these spiritual pathways within the Futhorc is a testament to the connection between the Pagan and esoteric Christian traditions; sometimes, and too often these are seen as being in conflict after this earlier era.

And here are further more specific runic associations to alchemy and the Grail:

Runes twenty-eight to thirty-one (Ior to Calc) have elemental features; being, water, earth, fire and air (as spirit), if looked at successively and with a little latitude. I would also like to look at an alternative ordering with Ior and Ear exchanging places and hence the elemental order being earth > water > fire > air. I am doing this because it happens to align with the subtle progression of the elements, if looked at from a ritual and/or alchemical perspective. These are loose associations maybe, but they are interesting and quite suggestive of undercurrents that are not readily visible.

The basis of alchemy is a process. In very simple terms, the so-called literal *Work* is the transformation of the base metal, lead, into a noble one, gold. There is a physical aspect to this, but it is the more psychospiritual aspects that have risen to prominence, most notably with Jung and some of his followers. This sees the transformation as being the purification and perfection of *man*, in the true spiritual sense of the word.

The first phase of this, the *Lesser Work*, is where the elements clearly feature. The raw material (of the personality; maybe Jung's concept of *shadow*) is contained, burnt, washed, the pure features identified and separated, then joined in a new and more evolved state of being characterised by the union of male and female in the individual personality. These stages are characterised by the elements, and these are clearly present in these four runes. Calc is notably an inverted Eolh - Ψ, and is referred to as a cup, or chalice. The inversion may represent the embodiment of spirit within matter; that is, the body.

The second phase is called the *Greater Work* and is more spiritual in orientation, in contrast to the more psychological or mental Lesser Work. The stages are considered to be putrefaction/fermentation, distillation and then coagulation. I should point out that that these seven stages are generally acknowledged, although consistent with the relative obscurity of alchemy and the probable intentional obfuscation, there are all sorts of permutations and numbers of stages, maybe as many as there were alchemists.

A simplification of the seven-stage process outlined here, is a four stage one, roughly correlating to those of the Lesser Work, and colour-coded. Called nigredo > albedo > citrinas > rubedo in Latin, the progression is black > white > yellow > red and encompasses the *Whole Work* that is both Lesser and Greater Works combined into one simplified proves. It is relatively easy to see an elemental association here, although the explanation of the colour red with air, or even fire as an alternative, would take us too far afield into the alchemical vaults for our current purposes.

If dealing with the Greater Work in the Futhorc, there are only two runes left... or are there? I wonder whether the so-called Double Calc or KK – ᛣ – may actually herald the conjunction of male and female that characterises the completion of the Lesser Work, and that the inverted Calc – ᛉ – may symbolise the immersion into the stage of fermentation, sometimes recognised as putrefaction initially, rather like the physical process itself (as in brewing). If this is the case, then one part of the riddle of the latter runes might have a tentative solution.

Gar – ᚷ – is a spear, and the mystical association with the chalice is strong, both in the Passion of Christianity and in the various Grail Legends, where they are incorporated into the ritual procession. I have put Gar here for a reason that I will come to shortly, but it is like a Double Calc without the central stave, maybe pure spirit minus the physical body? (Now I am being highly speculative.)

Stan – ᛜ – normally precedes Gar, but I have put the rune here at the end, because the *Philosopher's Stone* is the end point – the symbolic completion of the Work. There are a couple of other associations I would like to add, such as it is the stone from which the sword Excalibur is drawn in the Arthurian Legends. Also, Stan is like a 'completed' fourteenth rune, Peorth – ᛈ. Is Peorth the beginning of this process and hence misplaced in its common position? Does putting Stan at the end, indicate a deep feminine undercurrent to the process, as reflected in both the Arthurian and Grail Legends that has been usurped by putting Gar at the end?

How this applies to the Grail legends, I have hinted at, but will not pursue in any detail here. It is just that I firmly believe that the later runes of the Futhorc have alchemical significance, and that this theme is readily applicable to the Grail legends. In doing this, I am linking pre-Christian traditions with esoteric or mystical Christianity; something that has been done in other ways (mainly via the chalice), so my inquiry reinforces this. It also links mystical Christianity more firmly with the Pagan Tradition than does its exoteric or religious structure.

There are these questions, and more. As stated, they are speculative and a product of my fertile imagination. But that is the nature of this work; it is about some sort of psychic archaeology as well as being to establish life and future into a traditional process. This section alone could be the subject of a separate work; it is necessarily a bit disjointed and incomplete. But it does indicate the level of inquiry that the runes can raise, as well as indicating they are not a separate feature of historical and idle curiosity, but a vital thread in a living spiritual Tradition.

Two comments in these latter two paragraphs, "how this applies to the Grail legends, I have hinted at but will not pursue in any detail here", and "this section alone could be the subject of a separate work; it is necessarily a bit disjointed and incomplete", now appear somewhat prophetic. I originally wrote them a decade ago whilst immersed in the runes and alchemy, yet the association of these disciplines with the Grail seemed obvious and strong at the time, although I have not seen it commented on in anything to this degree.

Maybe this account is the "separate work" I referred to then, although it is not my intention to go any further with either the Futhorc or alchemy at this point, apart from a few relevant comments that have matured in the intervening period. Maybe also there is another work yet to come, where the deeper imagery in the entire Futhorc, hinted at with Eolh and Peorth, will be explored in an alchemical manner. And it is prophetically possible that I may be using this comment in that envisaged work... Presently, it is simply the case that I find these associations significant in this earlier period of time and not negated by an emerging Christianity that is largely of Pagan origins and hence inclusive of prior Tradition. Rather, I want to use this material to identify some of the themes I have yet to explore further, because they are all in there.

Sexuality and The Feminine

Gender and sexuality run through the Futhorc at various points, culminating in the extension with its alchemical and Grail associations, and even seen in the Procession Ritual itself. I will remark on these only inasmuch as they are contained in the major Grail theme, otherwise I will be exploring and defining what I essentially see as a kind of *Tantra of the West*. The gender and sexual themes are also apparent in the runes before the extension. Given that runes are, at one level, a kind of written language, this is hardly surprising; gender is rife in many languages, it seems Modern – not Old – English has been better than most of ridding itself of this (how 'English').

Beginning with the rune, Ior, and the comments above, this condensed and latently bisexual image becomes differentiated. Through the alchemical process inherent in the Northumbrian extension, the different components – genders – are variously alchemically separated and reunited. It won't surprise many if I were to say, following my 'Tantra of the West' comment, that alchemy used sexuality, between at least the alchemist and soror mystica, as a tool in their explorations. Embedded in the various medieval Grail poems are many edited sexual encounters; no wonder the Church needed to deal with this supposedly pernicious corpus.

The two ultimate images that emerge in the rune extension are the chalice and the spear, which in the medieval poems become the main icons in the Grail Procession. Not only is the actual physical nature of the Grail uncertain (chalice, dish, platter, stone…), but so is its form in the Futhorc when I wrestled earlier with the image for Calc. And maybe this also reflects a diversity in the feminine that various personages exemplify in the poems, as well. In contrast, the spear as Gar seems relatively straightforward; again, a feature of the male gender and its contrast with the female, although looks can sometimes be deceptive. In many ways Gar resembles Calc, and I am still a long way from reconciling these subtle differences and anomalies; indeed, if I ever can.

It is worth noting that the feminine features strongly in the Futhorc, and not just in a sexual manner. I suspect this reflects the more gender-balanced perspective of northern European cultures, Celtic and Teutonic specifically, where the status of women was acknowledged to be on a par with men; another reason for the Church to interfere. Even the first rune of the Futhorc is the feminine Feoh – ᚠ – which means something like wealth or possessions: Who really had the power, I wonder?

This pattern is not simply present in the runes that are, after all, a reflection of the society from which they emerged. The masculine and feminine balance of women and men in society was more egalitarian in these Pagan traditions. Although this may seem to be social and economic in a previously hunter-gatherer and early agricultural culture, it permeates their mythology, ritual and religious functions. In the Celtic Tradition women have almost an exalted role, if their mytho-religious organisation is considered. The destruction of this balance and hierarchy, with the advancement of the Iron Age and later Christianity with its patriarchal structure, may have a lot of do with the wounding of the King, and ultimately the Land, that emerges in the Grail legends.

If Nordic culture is taken as a background, although even this rests on a more shamanic culture, the gods and goddesses seem to have been in some kind of balanced relationship, unlike their Mediterranean counterparts. Ultimately, the god who emerged as pre-eminent in the first millennium is Odin who, in an apparently bellicose society, was noted for his gender ambivalence. Odin is a shamanic figure, who had the magical ability called in Old Norse *Galdr*, associated with the word and specifically poetry. Yet he also practised ON *Seidr*, which is a feminine magical art. He learned this from the goddess Freyja, who was also quite liberated sexually; in light of what precedes this, one wonders how he so learned...

It should not be forgotten that Odin and Woden are relatively synonymous; Odin has many different names, such as Wotan in Germany. Woden is even a desired person to have in your ancestral genealogy if you have aspirations to power, nobility and even kingship in the British Isles. And, as I have indicated, Merlin himself could be seen to be a latter-day reflection of this pre-Christian god. To this, I will return.

What has gone wrong here, that the Grail legends emerge to tell us of and maybe try to heal? Is this the most appropriate question for healing the Grail King? My contention is that the legends may show the patterns inherent in the wounding and healing, but this was truncated by the establishment – not just the Church – and the task is still there to do. Or maybe it is recurrent and these themes heal, but require renewal in successive eras. Or further, that with the advent of individuality, there is demand to do this intrapsychically on all our behalfs, as well as in the world of climate change and environmental fiascos, combined with the impending declines of both the Church and capitalism.

My dreams point to sexuality in the Childhood Dream, medicine in the Original Dream and religion in the Sacrificial Dream, or possibly all three together, because these are interwoven themes. They most definitely are in this account, and reflected in my Grail 'dreams'. These are the issues around which healing needs to be addressed. As I hold my dreams as a kind of psychic background, I can now look at the Grail material with the above questions in this section to mind.

What I see in the Grail Procession is the Lance and Grail as being central. The Sword, though also representing wounding, is more associated with Kingship, specifically that of the Grail or Fisher King. The blood on the Lance might be something other than this. The whole procession relates to the feminine with the Grail after the initial masculine entrance, where the bleeding Lance features. This Grail is one of plenty, referring both to a preceding era prior to the Iron Age maybe, when the Land was abundant and healthy, as well as being a symbol of death and resurrection, or an *elixir of life*; in fact, a condensation of many features symbolising much. No wonder then that it takes on a varied image, depending on which mythic aspect it is referring to. In this respect, Christianity referring to it as a Eucharistic Chalice is quite compatible; what is incompatible, is making it the *only* featured symbol.

In my dreams, I see that the original man is worn out and needs healing. The Grail in my hands in the dream is a jar that will need a vice to open it. I now suspect this is a balanced feminine aspect that I did not have at that age, though present in professional guise as my assistant, Julie. In the Sacrificial Dream the man is more wounded and his wounds are being inflicted by a giant pin or spear, by the masculine. It is not me that performs the healing here – maybe because in one way I *am* the man – this is performed by the feminine in magical guise. And I am the man because of the Dream Addendum I had recently, where he clearly now represents me.

What follows is speculative, although carries validity with my dreams being a representation of the mythic structure covered here. It appears that the masculine has been wounded in a sexual and regenerative way; he is not fertile. This wounding is self-inflicted because of a wound he identifies with; being the wounding of the feminine. This is his own inner femininity, woman in the world, and the Land. He must heal this to revitalise himself and the Land with him, but this healing is in the hands of the feminine.

It may well be that it is this generic 'man' that has inflicted the wound originally on the feminine and the Land. Maybe an accord has been broken and the primal unity sundered? The healing is about the restoration of his own masculinity and fertility through the agency of the feminine. He must repair this relationship, restore the balance. It is the agency of the feminine – both in the poems and in my Sacrificial Dream – that performs this. And I – we – present ourselves to her wounded and vulnerable, even unto death. Isn't she the agent of renewal here too?

The difference between the Sword and the Lance is significant. The Lance is more central and related to the feminine; it is healing at the psychosexual and psychospiritual levels, maybe one from the other. The healing of the Sword is the restoration of the Grail Kingship and the right of succession. In another view, the Lance is less gender inclined, as it is carried by a youth; in alchemy, this would represent an asexuality that approximates the hermaphrodite, but maybe here in balance after the wounding is healed. Recall that Odin had such a balance.

What I am saying here is not incompatible with other spiritual systems. In the Bible, it was the imbalance that led to Adam and Eve's ejection from the Garden of Eden. It was the violence of their sons that contributed to the ongoing, and our present state of the masculine. But I don't want to focus just on Christianity – these features are present elsewhere – it is just Christianity is familiar to many and having it symbolically and mythically decoded is the path to integrating it more holistically. The medieval attempt did not do this, at least to this point in time.

In Celtic mythology, maybe it is the accord with the feminine and hence the Land and the Faery realm that has been broken. Maybe this is because the masculine raped her (an interesting inversion of Eve's actions) and took the possessions, then to divide further amongst his kind in acts of power and vengeance. I am on thin territory here with my knowledge base, but someone like Joseph Campbell and his work reassures me that these deep patterns seep into the present; Jung with this archetypal theory would endorse this. I would like to take a particular approach to this that is compatible with both.

The symbolic connection to this unbroken mythic past invites us, in the present, to plumb the depths of our wounding to attain true healing, when in modernity we tend to gloss over or fix problems in a temporary manner. We don't travel into the wounding sufficiently or deeply enough to get to what we metaphorically refer to as the *core of the problem*.

The Grail Procession is an event quite different in tone to all the adventures in the Arthurian landscape that surrounds it; the Round Table and its symbology notwithstanding. The latter present a different image of the feminine and love in a courtly manner, which are more about tales with metaphoric and moral import, in contrast to the deep symbolism of the Procession. The icons that are present there include the Sword, Spear of Lance, and Grail, where the latter can be several things, although I incline to a Cup/Chalice and Cauldron, with a Stone being of alchemical import and synonymous with the Grail when it is considered as a unified image, as the *only* icon.

These icons have been paraded before, with the Tuatha Dé Danann in Irish mythology; they are the imported *Hallows* that subsequently became treasures and mirrored the socio-political organisation of Ireland. According to the history of invasions, it is considered that the Tuatha moved into the landscape with the coming of the Celts from central Europe that then followed, marking the beginning of the Iron Age, around 500 BCE.

Beyond the historical picture is the mythic one of a race from *Hyperborea* (beyond the North Wind), governed by a female goddess, Dana, who melted into the landscape and can still 'talk' from there. This is the Land of Faery, the mythic level of our being that accounts for phenomena such as changelings, sexual encounters between human and non-human forms (remember Merlin's conception), and all manner of things currently in the paranormal and supernatural category. It may also be the theme that the violence and vengeance of the Grail legends points toward.

In Hyperborea the Hallows, or consecrated icons, were contained within four cities that also marked the four compass points. Loosely applied and in the Southern Hemisphere, the Sword is in the East with the element of air; Spear or Lance in the North with the element of fire; Cup or Chalice in the West with water; Cauldron in the South with earth; and – if considered – the Stone at the Centre. I mention this because of the elemental associations and alchemical references, also because it is a mandala, therefore relating to the *self* of Jungian thought. (NB. Reverse the North and South in the Northern Hemisphere.)

These Hallows were brought to Ireland, but mythically to the Isles as a whole, and have progressively disappeared with the successive invasions; these being Celtic, and maybe latterly, the British. But it would be a mistake to assign these images and forces simply to Ireland, because there is a more extant and less plundered mythological tradition there; it could also be seen that this is a patten that exists elsewhere, maybe universally. No wonder the medieval Church was keen to appropriate the Grail legends.

The emergence of the Hallows in the Grail legends via various mythic, bardic and even runic pathways, I deem significant; although someone like Jung would see this as an inevitable return of repressed 'archetypal' material from the 'unconscious'. In the

Procession, the hallows come mainly via the feminine and return there, minus the Sword it is noted; although, interestingly, it is the feminine to where the Lance disappears too. They are, indirectly maybe, in the possession of the Grail or Fisher King and his female associates. The King is wounded, and it is the task of Parzival to heal him, but is this really with a question?

Here I am back to the forgetting:remembering dyad. As the Christian gloss is removed, I feel the failure to ask of the King the question as to what ails him goes with this dyad; it is based on guilt from various sources, though psychoanalytically his relationship with his mother. Instead, and in contrast to the already perfected Galahad, he is an innocent and naïve young man, who could not be expected to ask the question, even if his failure is condemned by others; this is simply part of the process, I would think. The 'process' is that he somehow should fail, then have to pass through the experiences and initiatory stages necessary to approach the King. Parzival must travel the Waste Land, encounter the challenges therein, die before he dies in a spiritual manner. There is a legacy there, a wife and family to which he will return after he has achieved his goal, fulfilled his destiny, become the Grail King. Viewed this way, the question is not the issue.

When I was not able to open the jar, I did not know what the vice was, I was not ready. But the dream and what I had somehow failed to achieve then haunted me. Following this dream, my career, previously on the apparent ascendent, seemed to collapse and with it family and financial gains. Yet it wasn't until I saw the wisdom in these apparent tragedies, reinforced by the Sacrificial Dream and subsequently facing my own near-death experiences, that I was able to approach the issue again.

During this period my values were reoriented. Remembering became remembrance, compassion the co-suffering born of empathy, and love became more multifaceted than I had previously know. Pain and suffering became more than trauma to be dealt with and forgotten, they became tools for my own healing and with it the re-evaluation of life and my wyrd; a discovery of soul.

The Question of Love

In this section, I am going to focus more broadly on values and issues like morality. This work is hardly a treatise on love, but the topic cannot be avoided. My position, therefore, is to see love as a superseding state of attainment in which more specific values are contained. This will be a generally idiosyncratic section representing some views from my personal experience that are consistent with and relate to the broad focus of the narrative.

As a medical doctor who spent most of his professional life working with both body and mind, ultimately as a holistic physician and medical psychotherapist, it is not surprising that I adopted my training's emphasis on the brain, even to seeing it as the repository of the mind. My psychospiritual explorations have caused me to turn a lot of this training on its head (pun intended) with respect to emphasis, at least. I have also liberated myself from what is essentially a solipsistic and cognitive worldview. In this view, the cognitive perspectives of reductionism, quantification, causality and dualism reign supreme, as the mind is seen as a product or even a by-product of the brain.

In the face of strong opposition in education and conditioning, my therapeutic work taught me that emotion is an all-pervading force that is far more powerful than the cognitive mind. I started to see that psychology and psychiatry were misnomers; they had little to do with the soul (Greek: Psyche = Soul) and were grounded in a cognitive framework. Mind you, medicine is far from alone. However, our inability to deal effectively with issues like cancer, infectious disease epidemics and serious mental health issues is increasingly obvious. As are the band-aid, fix-it types of approaches we adopt as management, which is often in conflict with and sometimes diametrically opposed to true healing. I have written about these issues extensively elsewhere, so here want to highlight the salient points as a kind of introduction to what will follow.

As discussed above, I have distinguished the cognitive mind from emotion, even seeing the latter as superior in value. In brief, self-aware responsible emotion leads to a discriminatory feeling capacity. As mind relates to brain via thinking, but is not a product of it, so soul relates to heart via feeling and is also not a product of it either. Instead, both brain and heart are contained in mind and soul respectively, and accessed through their thinking and feeling functions predominantly. The body forms a triad with these and spirit is the supervening fourth, so forming either a quaternary (as with Jung) or a hierarchal order (as in the perennial philosophy). In this reordering, mind contains the body, yet transcends it; soul contains the mind, yet transcends it; and spirit contains and supervenes them all. Hence my reasoning for equating the mature psychological self with the soul, when the inner realms are considered, which I believe Jung expands to include the transpersonal and spiritual realms with his rather unique concept of *the self.*

To gain a better perspective of values, more than cognition allows, it might be useful to consider some of the terms I have used to date and run them through this reordering process. As an aside, taking nouns and making them into verbs ('verbalising' them) takes us from structure to process; masculine to feminine; mind to soul. Also, the body can now be included beyond the stricture of mind, and so add another pathway to reconcile the body:mind conundrum.

Earlier, I took memory away from the exclusive noun to include a verb quality, as in *remember* or *remembering*. Remember is then not simply something forgotten, it is also something brought back into unity from a *forgotten* place; going to a noun via this route is remembrance. Remembrance is something we value, not simply the retrieval of something forgotten. Interestingly, remember also means to bring separated bodily members back together; a very concrete example of holism.

I am not going to go through a list of values and put them through this mental sieve; instead, it is something I do when I come across a similar conundrum that I had not previously considered. I also make sure I am using my feeling discriminatory functions, so that my heart and soul are engaged in the process. I recently did this here with *compassion*. Beyond looking at the term in verb and adjectival form, I also broke it down to com- and -passion; com- I took as *together*, and -passion, well, as *passion*. Passion is emotional, yet also erotic, or sexual, if the body is considered. But, and seemingly paradoxically, it is used to cover the events around and including the Crucifixion and Resurrection. So, passion can mean suffering? Well, it does in German, where compassion can indicate co-suffering, or empathy. It is an emotionally-loaded term; the heart needs to be engaged to fully appreciate it.

Yet another way of decoding values is to break them down in an etymological fashion, even if somewhat amateurish it can be easily done with a good dictionary. When this is done, it can be surprising what is revealed and what holistic connections made. Sometimes this is simply breaking the word down, as I have done above with *remember* and *compassion*. I even – somewhat cheekily – did it earlier with Lance-lot. When this is done the component syllables or words may reveal not only hidden English origins, or ones further afield like -passion in German, but also past origins (here a good dictionary is very, very useful); these are commonly French, Greek and Latin, but it is surprising how many have a Middle or Old English derivation.

It seems to me that other languages are often more emotive. We say this about the French, but really that language only arrived on the British doorstep just before the Grail legends, which were not primarily written in either French or English anyway. Maybe this is also because many foreign languages have gendered nouns, because the word *soul* has many more terms for it in German compared to English, and feminine ones at that. In a relatively trite way, maybe this explains the notorious English stiff upper lip and control of emotionality – as if that is possible. And, even if it were, the body suffers... says this doctor with experience. When Old English, the language of the Anglo-Saxons, is encountered in modern words, it always surprises me how they are both emotional in a raw way and embodied. It is no wonder that swear words and other terms with sexual innuendo have Old English as a foundation.

I mention all the above as it is a framework I employ when researching and writing. I find it emotionally challenging, creative, and rewarding. But now, with a little trepidation, on to love.

We, of the English-speaking world, have more or less adopted the Greek breakdown of love, being *Eros*, erotic or passionate love (although I question 'passion' here); *Philia*, love of friends and others of a sibling-like nature; *Storge*, love of parents for children (and maybe vice versa); and *Agape*, love of mankind, often used in a religious context. These are general definitions with a fair degree of overlap. Here, I would like to focus on Eros and Agape.

There is a term in spirituality-inclined psychologies named *spiritual bypass*, which is the *"tendency to use spiritual ideas and practices to sidestep or avoid facing unresolved emotional issues, psychological wounds, and unfinished developmental tasks," (John Welwood)*. These are as in Jung's *shadow*, or repressed material with a strong, dark and often traumatic emotional content. Something similar and often overlapping can occur with love, when the erotic and sexual tone of *eros* is conceived of as *agape* instead, to similarly avoid facing sexual and/or emotional undercurrents.

To Pagan cultures, such psychological manoeuvres were relatively unnecessary, as the boundaries of the sexual were not contained by a controlling religious structure making such sublimation a consequence. Rather, Pagan gods exhibit a full range of erotic and amorous activities, so the problem does not present itself; instead, such activities were often ritualised and used directly for spiritual experiences from a sexual source. The modern parallel in the East is Tantra, which the modern West lacks connection to; thus, so often and not always appropriately, importing techniques from Tantra wholesale. This is not usually compatible with western psychological sensibilities.

This difficulty with sexuality began to emerge in European culture early in the last millennium with the Church specifically, and the establishment generally, taking a suppressive attitude toward it. What emerged from this pattern was *Courtly Love* amongst the nobility; I am guessing most so-called common people didn't have any conflict, unless dictated to and spied upon. Courtly Love was an experience between eroticism and spiritual realisation, "a love at once illicit and morally elevating, passionate and disciplined, humiliating and exalting, human and transcendent" (Francis Newman); a quote that is in itself an attempt to unite the opposites of eros and agape or eros:agape.

Commonly conceived of as the love of a knight for a married lady, when the marriage was often considered an arrangement of convenience, this was, of course, adulterous in the eyes of the

Church should it be sexualised. Ideally and in theory, it was not and circumvented the religious police. In practice, of course it was. We have Lancelot and Guinevere with the cuckold King Arthur, and Tristan and Iseult with the equally hapless King Mark as literary examples, irrespective of the fact that both stem from deep Celtic mythic sources that carry different values, emphases and meanings in their behaviour and acts.

Courtly Love seems to be an attempt compatible with the religious, political and social values of the time to reconcile a tension in the eros:agape dynamic without conflicting with those same values, but maintaining a lifeline into Eros. It didn't work. Eros and its physical and emotional drivers are just too much for such control, as touched on a little earlier; it was – and is – doomed to fail. Maybe this is the fundamental flaw at the heart of Arthur's court.

As others have done, it may be of value to champion the Roman god *Amor* (amour). A parallel to Eros, Amor is seen in modernity more as providing the continuum between Eros and Agape; instead of either-or, it is both-and. So, the loved becomes the *beloved* in erotic, passionate and spiritual wholeness. Amor is a bridge between Eros and Agape, *devotion* extending from the beloved, synonymous with *consecration*. Eros:agape resolved and a spiritual pathway opened.

This discussion seems necessary to me, as it is a thorny problem that sits below the establishment in the hands of the poets, who are of bardic, troubadour or minnesinger disposition; they are all *love poets* with roots in their traditional and mythic pasts, prior to the social demands of their time. Excuse the pun, but they keep the flame burning. And the Grail poems are full of these sorts of issues. Perceval and Blancheflor in Chrétien spend amorous nights in each other's arms, but the issue of sexuality is not raised; indeed, academics to this day still argue whether they did actually *sleep* with each other in the way the euphemism inclines to.

In seeming contrast, Wolfram provides a picture of Parzival that fulfils a true vision of Courtly Love, although his future wife, Condwiramurs, is not married to another. Although she does become his wife, and devotedly so, she has her own standing and independence, so comes from a seemingly level playing field in this love match. Does the -*amur* part of her name signify *amour*? Parzival stays faithful to her vision in his adventures and ultimately wins both her and the Grail. Wolfram is here giving a more pre-Christian view of woman and her status, and one that is not primarily based on erotic dynamics; he is also skilled and adept at avoiding the censors, it seems, whilst also paying them homage.

What I am wrestling with here is that the Church took – and takes – particular aim at erotic love. There is a reason for this; rather like the centrality of the Grail and Lance that hardly require a symbolic interpretation, it is erotic sexuality that is the instinctual fire of evolution, initiation, transformation and spiritual realisation. No wonder the Church and establishment were – and still are – threatened. In the East, Tantra takes advantage of this pattern of personal evolution and exploits it. In the West, we have repressed it under the weight of trauma, guilt, obligation and fear.

The concept of amour is the poets' way of reconciling and creatively transforming the sexual instinct to the spiritual archetype; in brief, the other components of love do not have this power. Maybe this also adds a further level of meaning to the Fisher King's wound (and hence mine); one that seemingly Parzival transcends, so then not having to go through the same trauma as the Fisher King. In modern parlance, and because the Fisher King is also his uncle, he has broken a pattern of generational sexual trauma. Maybe that is what makes this poetry magnificent: Who needs modern psychology?

What emerges for me here about love is similar to my views about magic. Earlier in Part One, I discussed how magic was a kind of supervening principle that contained four or more tangible elements. In a similar manner, the various sub-components of love defined by Greek terms may collectively make up *love*. This, like magic, is a holistic perspective, where holism is more than the sum of the parts that go into making it. So, love contains the Greek components, but is also *more* than an aggregation of those parts. It is the opposite of reductionism, where in essence "we murder to dissect" (Wordsworth).

Courtly Love seems to be moving toward this, as it reconciles two components; or at least, tries to expand on eroticism to make it compatible with spiritual love, or *agape*. There are also other love components in the poems of a filial and familial kind. Collectively, they embrace all facets and make this true love poetry; the naming of such poets as the *minnesingers* as 'love singers' is therefore very appropriate.

Dreamtime

In shamanic terms, what I am undertaking here is a form of *soul retrieval* in both the individual and collective sense. One of my concerns is that at the world level, particularly in the West, we have lost our collective or world soul; the *anima mundi* in some schools of thought. My core thesis here is that the individual and collective levels of our existence resonate in a deep manner, with my own specific focus being on personal responsibility and intention. I see the individual soul being approached and becoming relatively synonymous with the wholesome psychological self, which has integrated its shadow; that is, a body, mind and heart unified.

Consequently, individual *retrieval work* becomes collective as well and thus approximates to Jung's ideas, particularly that of the shadow. It is simply that I see soul as a more relatable and hence attainable state of being, avoiding such issues as spiritual bypass remarked upon earlier, and then radiating out to the collective and spiritual realms. The place of suffering is significant and even central to this process.

To approach shamanism in a more holistic, integrated and modern manner, it may be useful to provide a mental picture of what I have been trying to create with my understanding of the Grail legends. Initially, it might seem that I am taking a non- or even anti-Christian stance. I have done this in the past, but I am making an attempt to make peace with this significant theme in my upbringing and life. Even though I now still stand outside the Church, I do not want to negate it or what it has meant to me. In appreciating the more esoteric and mystical aspects inherent in the legends, I have seen Christianity as one such theme mongst many. I have done thus by de-historicising and de-literalising the Christian stories around supposed events like the Passion, and placing them in a more mythic as well as appropriate cultural context.

With the Grail legends, the discussion has centred too often – and maybe too much – around a Christian versus Celtic argument. I consider now whether the Christian accretions to the core mythic structure are appropriate, but irrespectively, they are most certainly relative. The Celtic themes, to me, provide a continuity with antiquity that Christianity may provide in its Middle-Eastern context, but is more recently religiously grafted onto the Traditions it has superseded and then sought to appropriate. In effect, it is a dominating monotheistic cult not of our psychic heritage, which the Celtic structure, with its less military religiosity, tends not to be. So, in establishing itself, Christianity has also suppressed and hence obscured; maybe and simply because it is culturally insecure.

By looking at the runes and the context in which they emerged, I have found that, prior to Christianity becoming so much a doctrinaire and establishment tool, it was connected with imagery of a more magical nature even within its own ranks. I suspect this continuity became disrupted and that, in Jungian fashion, the Grail legends emerged as a compensating collective demand for psychological balance, only for them to be – somewhat severely – suppressed again by the Church and the ensuing Inquisition. The irony here, is that the life of Jesus, and the stories around it, may themselves have represented a similar uprising over a thousand years prior. The realisation here is that such events occur periodically as a spiritual imperative, when the religious structure, that contain its cultural myths, become controlling and decadent with a power imperative, making them somewhat synonymous with what I have periodically referred to as the *establishment*.

Interestingly in modernity, the loss of the Church's power and control has seen the rise of other collective structures to assume that position. As an example, one of the most significant is science in the general sense. Having been a tool of inquiry, it has now attracted a belief system – to deal with our fears – in a manner analogous to the Church and with it has taken on a religious veneer: Science as *scientism*. In my own field of psychospiritual medicine, I have seen the breakthroughs and insights of the likes of Freud, Adler, Jung and Reich subsumed into or suppressed by establishment medicine and psychology, their 'movements' already ossified, intellectualised and tools of the said establishment. Following the recent pandemic (in 2020), maybe this compensating imperative is to be found in other areas and disciplines, as re-emerge it must and will; that is one clear message of the Grail legends, as well as being a psychological truth.

Within the legends themselves, this is what attracted me first to Geoffrey of Monmouth and Merlin, which I thought would be my route into the inquiry I was undertaking. Then I was drawn into and started looking at Perceval in more detail, and hence Chrétien's work. But latterly it is Wolfram who attracted me, as his Parzival was embedded in a greater vision that included the East and alchemy. It was essentially a more holistic work, and one I am sure I will be returning to in the future. It holds a visionary and spiritual beacon, in my view.

Yet, in this summary account of my endeavours to date, I have not lost sight of Merlin and will seek to place him in some kind of relationship to Parzival. This is because I have been drawn back into patterns, displayed in such myths as the Tuatha from Hyperborea, in the magical and shamanic world from which Merlin emerged. It is these patterns that I believe need more clearly resurrecting in the modern world; we need to go back to move forward. We also need to see this past, and even the future it points to, in the present. My belief is it is concerned around life and death, wounding and healing, sex and power, where this pattern – the lost Grail – hovers and oscillates.

Here in Australia, I have a clearer view of this process, realising how any archeologically-inclined psychic 'dig' could only go so far. In a practical sense, this is because the difference in Australia between the colonisers two hundred years ago and the indigenous peoples is a rift that spans many, many thousands of years. I watch the paradox that it is the controlling establishment trying to undertake a so-called healing, when they are instead simply using the Church's method of divide and conquer to retain power. This means that the indigenous culture has a lot of catching up to do to be sufficiently enabled to deal with this pattern. The flaw being, of course, that they may never be experienced enough to deal with the establishment on its own terms and the dualistic and oppositional dance continues on the invaders' terms.

Instead, we should be looking to the animistic culture on its own terms and see how it offers solutions to environmental, economic and political problems that the establishment has both generated and perpetuated. Because this establishment is on insecure ground, like the Church before it, as the process is based on power and appropriation, which happens to the degree that they are both progressively disconnected from their mythic basis and hence spirit; that is, it is insecure and psychically disempowered. These psychic divisions are palpable wounds and such patchwork and controlling 'healing' is no healing at all. We are creating a wasteland and are dying in the consequences, when around us are the means of healing. But this requires a shamanic sensibility, one that listens to the myth and spirituality born of these many, many thousands of years occupancy, enshrined in mutual care and sustainability: Are we ready to listen?

And what is this 'shamanic sensibility'? Although I have discussed this in some detail earlier in Part One, it may be useful to encapsulate it. Central to it is the concept of soul, which can be either lost or possessed, dim reflections of which are seen in the anachronistic but still useful psychiatric concepts of neurosis and psychosis respectively. The person with a lost soul is psychically divided, without personal power and subject to illness, both mental and physical. In passing, it suits the establishment when it is collectively divided from its mythic and spiritual foundations to keep people in this state. The Church does this by alienating us from such forces as sexuality, and the establishment through other channels, such as medicine and its state-sanctioned controls. A person becomes possessed when these divisions facilitate the forces of the spiritual collective to engage them in a manner in which they have no control, either because divided as in soul loss, or because the necessary powers of self-control have not been developed. Remember, all spiritual forces are as Jung's archetypes, latently bipolar and inherently powerful; they can be dark, dangerous and evil when disowned and projected. A psychically divided collective establishment is not immune from this pattern, as recent twentieth century history adequately portrays.

A shaman is able to separate from the affairs of the world and enter a liminal state through ritual process. In this state, they may simply undertake contact with the world of spirit in a trance, charmed or enchanted state, and mediate this in an artistic, healing or poetic manner. This is referred to as *divination*, where the shaman does not lose control of the individual self. If the world of spirit in actively engaged, the shaman may enter into it and engage with the archetypal forces there. The shaman has a mythic map for this purpose to help negotiate this risky and potentially dangerous territory. There may go the great artists and healers, retrieving ideas, images and even the souls of those lost to restore the balance of the world.

In Australia, this world of spirit is referred to as the *Dreamtime*. The relationship of the daily world of men in their journeys between birth and death is in balance and sustained by ritual and ceremony. This ritual is not just for shamans, it is for all and is an integral part of initiation that includes sacrifice; no change will occur without this. Ceremony is where others in community participate in the connection through dance, song, art and word. Axiomatic to this, is that the health of the world is maintained, sustained and healed, when necessary, by this dynamic relationship between the worlds by individual, tribe and the broader community. The relationship extends to how the individual conducts themselves in the world and is reinforced by such forces as law and taboo grounded in collective myth for the welfare of all; it is easy to see how this can be manipulated and abused.

In European culture, the King emerges as the repository of such values. And with the challenges and mixed blessings of progress, the checks and balances were in the hands of religious authority, be it the shaman or, in Britain his Druid successor. This balance between Church and State is ideally balanced and dynamic, not separate. The boons of this contract with spirit and its reflection in the world are the gifts that can be seen in the images of the Hallows, and specifically the Grail; here a symbol of this relationship and its unity. If the image is lost, as with an imbalanced or ill King or the abuse of power, rectification is sought with mythic guidance. The storehouse of memory, story and myth increases over time to engage in this manner. Should the relationship be seriously damaged, the world suffers; it becomes a Waste Land. This is particularly so if we rape it – or her – as is our current predicament. Aboriginal people maintain this primal balance in a way we invaders have lost touch with;

should we restore this balance in cooperation with them and not continue our rapacious and disordered ways in politics, medicine and the environment, a new order will emerge: The Grail revisioned; a beacon to the world.

It is our stories that tell us this. The Passion is one such story, the Grail another. We are searching for a story of our time; *Lord of the Rings* is one such attempt. Our actions also talk to us; the story of the 20thC politically was not good, as medicine and the environment lurch lemming-like to an unclear misty precipice. We believe such restoration is in our scientific hands, but without the guidance of spirit and a new story, it is not. Or if it is, it is more in the hands of our artists, storytellers and shamans… it is in the hands of individuals, not companies, professions or the state. It requires the balance between the individual quest to restore one's own and their obligation to community; a delicate balance not unlike a tightrope… or the edge of a sword.

To end this section, I would like to draw on two experiences from Aboriginal culture that reinforce what has been expressed above. They also point to the unseen depths that exist, lest we are drawn to much in seeing our comparatively recent historical stories – both mythic and historical – in some sort of isolated, elevated and even arrogant sensibility. The first I came across on an ocean trail in the Southwest at this point in my writing of this account:

Korrianne Gnwirri

> Korrianne was promised through Wadandi Lore to Datton, but she was in love with a strong young hunter, Medinite. She knew that soon she would have to leave, even though her *korda*, her heart, belonged to Medinite.

Korrianne would walk to the beach, collecting wildflowers and coloured shells. She would sit and weave some of them into her hair.

Medinite would hide close by, whispering: "Korrianne, Korrianne you are beautiful. Your eyes shine like stars, your skin is smooth, your hands are soft, your feet are strong. Beautiful Korrianne with the beautiful face... "

Soon Datton sent for Korrianne. She walked along the river, crying out loud, "Medinite, I'm so sad, so sad, my heart is sick. Medinite, I will die."

Korrianne soon left and Medinite stopped eating. Sadly, he soon died. Korrianne, the beautiful, also gave up and let the Great Spirit come and take her to *Kurranup*, where she still waits to be united with Medinite.

She sits weaving shells in her hair... waiting...waiting...for their hearts and souls to be united forever.

There are resonances here with the legend of Tristan and Iseult, married to Mark, as well as that of Lancelot, Guinevere and Arthur. There are reflections on Courtly love and the conflict of duty, lore and obligation, against individual desire. There is the prominence of the heart and the role of spirit. Some even peeks into the Grail Procession... the beauty, the coiffured hair. This is from a culture with a tradition that goes back tens of thousands of years. It puts the stories I have been relating into a deeper and more archetypal perspective, to my way of thinking... and feeling.

The second is less an experience than a known fact. In Aboriginal culture there is a punishment called *spearing* for transgressive acts against tribal lore. These may, for example, be stealing, or sexual transgression of a taboo. The punishment is called *payback*, as in revenge, but intended to restore balance in the community. The act is that a spear is thrust through, usually, the thigh and that is the end of the punishment. Obviously, death can occur depending on what is severed, and the recipient remains marked, or scarred. Yet there is wounding and healing embedded here, wounding:healing.

What intrigues me is that like the story of Korrianne, there is a conflict here between desire and duty or lore. What further intrigues me is the use of the spear and the inevitable blooding. We may be given to think that the Lance in the Passion and Grail legends is something more historically recent, but here it is stretching back many thousands of years into an animistic hunter-gatherer culture.

Doesn't this all just put this account into a far greater perspective?

Healing

I have entitled this section *Healing* as I would like to draw the relevant strands of this account together into some sort of whole, although as with all narratives, the journey will continue on. One imperative of this narrative is that I have chosen to weave my own individual story into it as one foundation, primarily through the dreaming process. This is by way of a personal *soul retrieval* as a testament of how the apparent template (fate, destiny, *wyrd*) of my life revealed and reveals itself in me through dreams, as well as other associated psychic and shamanically-inclined tools, which unashamedly includes my intellect. Because by now it can be appreciated that the intellect – in contrast to the cognitive mind – is also such a spiritual tool.

I have used this personal framework to explore the desire within me to understand my life's journey in a way that is inclusive of the more immediate personal story, but then radiated out into a larger social and cultural context, which itself is reflected here in many ways, including myths and creative products that feel to have relevance for me. What I have deduced from this is that the personal and meta- or transpersonal stories relate in some kind of fundamentally harmonic manner. This account has served to confirm this for me. I can and have, to some extent abstracted from this, including referring to others and most notably Jung, who did something similar. But I wanted to do this *my own way* and include my personal story directly: I believe this is important and too often omitted or neglected.

The outcome of this is an account that includes a personal journey. It has qualities of Campbell's *Hero* archetype in it, in that

I have acknowledged, but relatively eschewed, a life path directed by duty and obligation. But I did not want this to appear primarily iconoclastic, although the process that has arrived at this point has its full share of sabotage and trauma. And this is because I see trauma – wounding – as central to this individuation process; something modernity seems to have lost sight of. Also, this journey does not have a conclusion. In a personal sense, I may be drawing to the close of my life journey with the attendant imperative to make sense of it and put it into some sort of conclusion, as into a filing cabinet – or a book.

But this book does not simply take account of my personal journey. It flows back out into the transpersonal or collective in some sort of pattern that is better represented by the eternity glyph, a mobius strip, or the Yin-Yang symbol of the East. So, from here there will be loose ends and themes of relative incompleteness. Maybe they will become more complete in the future, left for others to do, or remain unfinished; spirit will determine this. Instead, I will now use *Healing* as the overarching theme in which to put some-but-not-all of what has preceded it, and then move into a futuristic gaze. Strap up.

Wounding

In a cumulative way, it must be readily apparent that I do not take a conventional scientific or medical view toward wounding. In a nutshell, I see that we are born into life within genetically appreciated family, heritage and ancestral patterns, into which our individual existence is inextricably woven; this is essentially a traumatic process and that we are wounded by life, we suffer it. The challenge of life, it seems to me, is the manner in which we negotiate trauma and wounding and how much we relate it directly to the creation or maturation of the soul.

This is not a pessimistic worldview, it is simply a just-so story of our existence; it is existential, but it is also humanistic. The trick seems to be how we make sense of our wounding, appreciating its fateful nature and where it is directing us. This demands an intrapsychic perspective, where projected issues like blame, guilt and fear ultimately simply avoid the central issue; what is the wounding telling me? This is why I see wounding as an integral component to soul-making, and what is demanded of me is to make sense of it.

In this way wounding has a spiritual component; it is directive in that it is providing meaning and purpose in a manner that we must appreciate, if we but have or find the necessary tools. To my understanding, this demands a disposition that is available to the symbolic and its images and ideas; a metaphoric appreciation of life; the ability to see analogy; and to appreciate humour. In other words, the capacity to embrace depth. This manner of looking at trauma is sometimes called the *divine wound*, being the wound that guides us to healing.

A shamanic sensibility appreciates this. I have slowly grown to appreciate and understand this in my own professional and personal life journey. It is also probably why I was attracted to the profession I was, to ascend the perennial worldview from body to mind, soul to spirit, through the wounding and trauma I saw in my patients and experienced in myself. I have also come to realise that this embraces concepts like the *dark night of the soul* as espoused by the Christian mystic, Saint John of the Cross, or the *night sea journey* seen as archetypal by the likes of Jung, where the individual, as hero, descends into the underworld and faces death in the path of individuation.

In shamanic terms, this can be likened to *soul retrieval* and it is synonymous with psychically entering into the wounding process or traumatic state to bring back to awareness that which is metaphorically lost, being the soul. Spirit governs this process and floods us with symbols and signs to assist us, though we must discern the source, because the darkness contains not only the light, but other forces and beings that would thwart us on our journey.

A template stands behind my story. There was a brother I never personally knew, who was sacrificed before term and interred on a family farm, as the instinctual drives of the couple concerned – my parents – had resulted in a culturally and socially unacceptable outcome. In this atmosphere of trauma and guilt I was later conceived, though I sense within myself somewhat reluctantly, and equally reluctantly delivered into an atmosphere of drugs and alcohol that had also embraced my bother in his passing. This pattern of events enveloped me and my upbringing. The traumas of my life have been a reflection of myself as inadequate, insecure, a replacement for *another*, but also a pathway back to this unravelling and understanding so that I could move forward purposefully and with clear intent. In effect, I am the resurrection of my brother, and hence myself.

My story is far from unusual and pales into insignificance compared with the challenges of many, yet is mine to walk and provides me an insight and empathy for the journey of others. It made me successful in my trade, although my profession wanted me not. And even as I write this, I see my pattern as that of everyman, but also to contain the symbolic and mythic icons in our collective story that embody these principles and point the way.

Although rich in significance for me, the path of Jesus as espoused by the Christian institution that followed in his name is not mine. Yet it also is, in that it is one amongst others, although in the 'others' there are ones that are closer to my heart. And this has been part of my retrieval process and which this account is testament to.

The Great Cycle of Existence

Alternatively seen as birth-sex-death-rebirth, this cycle was described earlier. It is what defines our existence in the world, our life or lives. Yet there are figures in supposed history and certainly myth who have sidestepped some-if-not-all of these seemingly inevitable steps. Jesus had a mixed birth, avoided sex (supposedly) and defeated death. This puts him *outside* of existence, at least relatively, which is not the same as being dead or non-existent. The focus, instead, is on wounding and portended death, which I have interpreted as a self-sacrifice. A question for me is whether his place outside existence was pre-ordained or a consequence of his self-sacrifice, then the story backfilled with mythic intelligence?

Merlin is somewhat similar, in spite of the Church's attempts to concretise him into a sexual liaison and deathlike entrapment with the likes of a Morgana. His mythic origins reside around the earlier figure of supposed history dealing with Vortigern, somewhere in the Southwest of Britain and Wales associated with other mythic themes, like Avalon. His negotiation of death takes us into the realms of magic and prophesy, as does the alternative figure of him in the North, although somewhat mythologised by Geoffrey and his death not elucidated; the inference being it might not have happened. Yet the triple death says otherwise, unless, of course, this is mythic and symbolic, rather like the Tarot equivalent or as a reflection of the Crucifixion. As a religious man, I still wonder how much of Geoffrey's work was more deeply influenced by the Church than I have appreciated.

Shamans have similar attributes, because they lead a marginal or liminal existence that is the consequence of their wounding and initiation experiences. The soul position that liminality describes is maybe a key here: Does this confer on the individual an access to the beyond that renders him or her immune from death as non-existence? Does the life of the shaman attract the mythic elements that render them partially or completely beyond the Great Cycle? How much is Jesus a shaman? Other questions follow…

Yet maybe this is why I was and am attracted to Merlin. I am trying to make sense of my own life journey and he emerged as an image, a guide in my childhood, and usurped the place of the Church's Christ. Merlin is somehow more accessible to the questions I have, or more culturally immediate. In this manner he hovers behind and imbues my dreams and my work without actually appearing in them. This is probably because his shamanic qualities show through more clearly, and resonate with – or directed – my choice to become a doctor. It may also be why I am attracted to magic.

Parzival

Yet my dreams relate more to the various stories of Parzival and his namesakes, and others, such as Gawain, Bors, Lancelot and Galahad. If I take the position of Parzival in my dreams, then the Fisher King is portrayed before me and I am directly (in the Original Dream) or indirectly (via the Witch of the Sacrificial Dream) involved in his healing. Yet in my life, I feel more the King and wonder whether I see Parzival more in my offspring, my sons, and that there is some sort of generational pattern here that I have to retrieve into myself? To my way of thinking, I must remain as Parzival, otherwise I am destined to continue wounded and in pain.

The distressed response to the entrance of the Lance in Wolfram's poetic Grail Procession is significant. It clearly indicates wounding and trauma, but of what nature? As one of the Hallows that also backfills even the Passion, it is deeply symbolic, reinforced by its presence and role in Aboriginal lore. It is tempting to see it sexually, which I will do, but with the caveat that this is in the context of the Great Cycle of birth-sex-death-rebirth (or resurrection).

The Lance is masculine like the Sword and represents a distinct singular phallic representation, but unlike the Sword, which with the scabbard is more related to sexual intercourse. In Wolfram, the blood emerges from the tip as semen would from a penis, the way it is held by the youth with the blood dripping into his sleeve is distinctly masturbatory. It is self-centred and not directed to another. I view this as a disconnected masculinity in the context of the Procession, maybe relating to violence, sexual abuse and vengeance. In a broader context, does this represent the actions of a warrior culture toward a more balanced one, a patriarchal dominance of the feminine elements that I have highlighted in many northern, pre-Christian cultures?

I believe so. In my Sacrificial Dream there is a representation of this, somewhat as happened to Jesus with the mythic centurion spear, maybe because he was also championing a transition. Is this what is happening to the man in the dream? At this stage in his ministry, Jesus had just had his feet anointed by a woman – maybe Mary Magdalene – and the resurrection provides a contrasting image of his complex and deep relationship with the feminine. Is this why the man in the dream is being punished, maybe executed? How far was Merlin also drawn into this drama?

The contrast is with the Sword at the conclusion of the Procession. It has a fault, known to its maker, that would break it again. In *Excalibur* it was Arthur's pride, but I doubt it here. I suspect before the final battle, when Guinevere returns the sword to Arthur, she is restoring the balance and his right of Kingship, after he discarded it on discovery of her tryst with Lancelot… and inadvertently brought about Merlin's apparent demise. She is returning his masculinity to him and it is covered in a cloth, maybe a reference to the scabbard, or a shroud, or even the membranes that sustain a child in the womb… the son they never had?

This is somewhat similar to Parzival and with it the right of Kingship, but in this case it is the Kingship of the Grail; it is a spiritual attainment, a different Kingdom. Yet the potential for it to break if the fault is re-enacted indicates something deep about wounding and well known in shamanism: We heal from our wounds but we retain the scars. Should we regress and not face the ongoing challenges that our healing directs us toward, then we can relapse. In the circumstance of Parzival, it requires he undergoes levels of initiation before he can return and attain the Grail, his innocence and lack of life experience renders this impossible on the first occasion he sees it and the suffering continues.

These events bookend the actual appearance of the Grail. They do in *Excalibur*, as Arthur is wounded with the symbolic lightening 'lance' in the Church before being healed by the Grail, after which the sword is returned to him to redress the faults and imbalances that his reign has produced and which Mordred symbolically represents. Ironically Mordred uses a spear to wound Arthur – again – yet the task is completed and, Christlike, Arthur goes to Avalon in the company of women, to be healed and potentially resurrected. Such is the stuff of myth; it embraces us still.

The Grail and Beyond

The elaborate and ritualised events in Wolfram are at one level a continuation of Chrétien, in that the cycle of Parzival's journey and return is completed, but he significantly adds a depth not present before. In contrast, Chrétien's other continuers, maybe with the notable exception of the *Elucidation*, provide an increasingly refined path into Christianity that was obviously in need of revival, although it is questionable to me whether this was achieved; in fact I think not, it seems 'business as usual'.

At the very core, this is a feminine mystery that is being revealed to the men present by the women who conduct a ritual in a ceremonial fashion. It is of interest that the women are described with flowers, a reference to garden, nature and the *Land*, whilst the blond hair may represent the Celtic or similar cultures and their Traditions that have been superseded by this masculine patriarchy. This seems a subtle reference to me of what Wolfram is trying to portray; elsewhere he indicates the connection of East and West, here it is the masculine and feminine maybe beyond the institutional systems of his time.

The Grail is pictured exclusively as a green stone by many commentators. If so, it is analogous to the stone of my Original Dream, which also emerges upon and behind the masculinised fountain. This latter feature, in and of itself, could point to the masculine usurpation and corruption of a feminine domain, the fountain. Other commentators make reference to the stone being alchemical; certainly, there are alchemical features in Wolfram, but I am unsure here. The stone is also one of the Hallows, and in this scene there is one – a red garnet – that makes the table on which the Grail is laid by its Queen. Her presentation of the Grail on the table in this manner reminds me of Guinevere's presentation of Excalibur to Arthur, but also the presentation of the baby Arthur to Uther... and hence Merlin. These resonances may not have been the writers' intent, but they are valid in an archetypal way.

Yet I wonder if the Grail is a stone? Although it is not clearly described as any sort of eating or drinking vessel, which themselves point back beyond the Jesus story to the patterns in many other cultures, including the Celtic. My impression is that it is obscured as an image, maybe deliberately so by Wolfram, to emphasise the numinosity of the witnessing experience prior to the image; this is in acute contrast to the distress that accompanied the Lance. Yet, taken as a whole, the ritual process to date is not unlike a conception and birth pattern.

At one level, transgression – particularly sexual – is quintessentially human. As is the challenge and breaking of taboo. I suspect the issue is with what intent it is entertained; if unawares, it is prey to dark intrusion and maybe this is what has happened here in the depths of our own history and beyond. And it is myth, even as represented by the poets and reflected from humanity's storehouse in my own dreams, which serve to remind us that such acts are to be undertaken with awareness and clear intent. At the core of this is the Great Cycle of Existence, and how we handle it, because we can't avoid it – try as hard as the Church has to do this and so to disenfranchise or disempower us.

There is a deep pattern in the Grail legends and it is reflected in the Hallows of the Tuatha, and makes its way into history with the runes and the Tarot in the context of our mythic past. Because this past is not history, it is ever-present: Consider such controversies as the struggle over the Stone of Scone as witness to this. The stone of the Hallows may be the foundation, and I will put it in the South (here in the Southern Hemisphere). It could also be seen as the centre, the paradox and ambiguity of which I will leave presently. It is the archetypal feminine, from which all things originate, including the Land in which we live and thrive.

The Lance is the contrasting archetypal masculine in the North. The blood is the sacrifice that the masculine undertakes to enter into the mystery of the feminine. The Grail is the product of their union, the archetypal genderless child of alchemy, the presence of spirit in the world. (NB. As before, swap the North and South if in the Northern Hemisphere.)

The Sword and the Chalice-as-Grail are the East and West respectively, like their transpersonal parents, they are anchored in the landscape. These are the King and Queen in the World, whose purpose is a balance union and with it the welfare and health of the Land and the people who inhabit it. Am I but describing a Garden of Eden myth here? Somewhat, but I am putting it into a distinctly culturally relevant context and one that we may more readily relate to than the Middle-Eastern one that we are commonly presented with.

The whole complex of the feminine and masculine, sex and power, death and renewal is writ large here.

The Return of Merlin

Embedded in Geoffrey's *History* is the short work called *The Prophecies of Merlin*, which was an independent work that he chose to embed in *History*. I wonder why. Maybe it was because *History* would be a bestseller of its time and carry the *Prophesies* forward with a momentum that would otherwise not have occurred; this remains a matter of speculation, but relatively unimportant. The fact is, the *Prophecies* exist.

When looked at in this way, collectively there is a body of work around this period that rivals not only the New Testament, but also the Old with its prophets and their Biblical prophecies. Maybe the fact that all this material was committed to writing guaranteed their temporal, political and religious success, which the likes of Geoffrey challenged… and from the inside. I suspect this collectively flew in the face of the Church and indicates a deeper spiritual drive than even the contemporary Crusades and the subsequent Inquisition, with their respective motives.

I am referring to Merlin as not only a mythic figure, but as a central archetype challenging Jung's *self*, which he identified in Jesus, as Christ. Merlin's heritage portrays the similarity, yet he comes in the tradition of others, such as the Welsh *Gwyddion* and the Nordic *Odin*. In so many ways I actually see Merlin more clearly as *Woden*. But these are semantics, the importance is his presence in whatever shapeshifting guise he chooses. Irrespective, in this manner I see him as a *Christ*, if that terminology be favoured, and hence a representation of the *Father*, as in the Allfather of the Norse Woden. Anyway, this is how I presently see him…

Prophecies is an obscure work. Maybe the product of Geoffrey's fertile and fevered mind, it carries weight to the image of Merlin, and is a tradition furthered by the likes of Nostradamus and William Blake. Prophecies takes the material of *History* and *Vita* into astrological territory and deeply reflects the alchemical features in Geoffrey and others, most notably Wolfram and reflected in Dante. I do not intend to go into any further detail here, I am not equipped to do so beyond putting it in context; but I felt to add it in, to point to the relevance and importance of astrology – it heralded Jesus' birth after all – as a complement to and extension of alchemy, and a spiritual representation of us and the Land at a cosmic level, as well as pointing out that trivialising Merlin as pointed-hatted and star-gowned magician belittles him and what he has to tell us. He tells us much; he is the inspiration behind this work.

With *Prophecies* Merlin paints an astrological symbolic view of the future. I suspect that their content is not only about the events of Geoffrey's time and the issues from history and mythology that he was resurrecting for that present and potential future, but also point to our time. Why? Because I believe we are at a transition point that I have identified as then too, as well as prior to the advent of Christianity in Britain. I identify it in our present world, with its spiritual bereft-ness, obvious degradation of the Land in the form of poisoning, and our contribution to issues such as Climate Change.

I further believe – know – that the recent Pandemic is part of this picture. Medicine joins religion in its contemporary irrelevance as we seek in science and technology solutions to the present impasse. It will prove to no avail, because it does not embrace magic and healing. We also – must – deal with our shadows, individually and collectively, and in that order. Our intelligence needs reconnection to heart and soul and then listen to spirit in our dreams and other portents. Many are doing thus; this work is simply a contribution to that collective pool.

Merlin wields magic in prophecy, healing and deed: Another reflection of Jesus. His magic is sympathetic to nature and heals transgression in a homeopathic manner. (Although his magical involvement in the begetting of Arthur does continue to haunt me somewhat; maybe a task for our time?) This is the deep feature of healing that homoeopathy grasps; it is what wounds us that also heals us. Our transgressions are our healing too. This homeopathic influence is deeply impressed in the symbolism of the Lance in the Procession. The sympathetic magic of Fraser and Weston is seen in the fertility rituals that stand behind those of the Grail and the mythic stories associated with Merlin.

It is this that provides a wholeness of interconnected parts to this narrative; not some sort of rational and simply intellectual analysis and reconstitution, but a healing by bringing the various parts together and realising in the aggregation that something more is born of this process. This involves our participation and in this way even miracles can be seen as sanitised magic. Merlin has done his job.

Sacrifice and Healing

> *I am watching a man who is making a concoction or kind of tincture. It is blood and organic matter from a dragon, that is diluted and put into a phial. There is someone else before him, seated or kneeling; he inserts the phial into the second man's mouth and empties some of the content in. I see the watery redness and some organic matter in it. Either I am next for this process, or it is me he is giving this to, as the insertion is very graphic.*
>
> *(Healing Dream)*

As with the earlier Addendum dream, I am bringing this very recent dream into this account. I had earlier determined to do this if anything I dreamed or experienced, whilst undertaking this writing, felt directly relevant; this most certainly does. Prior to having this dream, I was intending to return directly to the Sacrificial Dream; it seems spirit is both assisting and directing me away and further.

I relate the man and the tincture back to the jar of the Original Dream. Now I see what is in or being made in it, maybe related to both any blood spilled and the fluid in the Witch's potion in the Sacrificial Dream. The dragon, of course, takes me not only to *Excalibur* but more significantly to the Charm of Making and specifically the *Dragon's breath*. The breath is, of course, inspiration. However, I do see the tincture as a magical extension of this and the magician to represent Merlin.

The organic matter could be several things. In the context of the dream and the overall sequence to date, including this narrative, I see it as being similar to foetal material, or stem cells in the modern scientific vernacular. This puts the phial in Grail territory, as if the jar in its previous representations had not pointed that way enough already. This would make the liquid rejuvenative in essence, along the lines of an elixir, Bergson's *élan vital*, or the *elixir of life*.

> *Dragon's breath,*
> *the charm of death and life,*
> *thy omen of making.*

Something that has always intrigued me is the inversion of the commonly used phrase *life and death* to *death and life*. But am I reading too much into this? So, here's a little wordplay; a magical exposé.

I suspect the phrase in the Charm is deliberately inverted. If the Great Cycle is seen as life-death, or birth, sex and death in this existence, then the inversion points to or is reflective of the world beyond, the spiritual reality. *Thy omen of making* is then a spiritual conception, such that Merlin was attempting to ordain in Arthur's physical equivalent.

Yet this points to more; it is our own renewal, each and every one of us. It is why Parzival had two visits to the Grail castle and we also have to. It is what the mystics talk about when they refer to *dying before you die*, or the rebirth in spiritual tradition advocated in so many cults and regions, even the Christian one.

The journey for me, and this narrative that reflects it, is a magical act to attain this. It is a journey we all have the opportunity to undertake.

Epilogue

Merlin and the Grail in the Psyche

In my various researches, I have come to some sort of resolution about how I see Merlin in the world of history, mythology and spirituality. He is Geoffrey's creation and relates to the historical figure of Myrddin that is creatively elaborated in *Vita*. That Geoffrey originally chose to identify him with more mythic child in *History* intrigues me, as Nennius and others take that prophetic figure back into a more distinctly Welsh background, maybe even to the godlike magician, Gwyddion. Maybe this was a pretext for the *Prophecies* by having them uttered by one from a prior Celtic era.

I have scratched my head over this and, just as I was finally editing this work and wondering where I should go next, the figure of Faust came to mind with his potential and more magical association with Merlin. This was because my head-scratching was honing in on the Faust story – particularly as expressed by Goethe – as the next creative step of a fictional nature. But the association with Merlin precluded any furtherance of this step and led me back to this work, and specifically Merlin.

I dug around the mythic story of the prophetic youth further and intuitively settled on the – in my opinion – much vilified Vortigern. I was aghast to find that he had numerous children, but specifically three sons, then a (Jungian?) fourth, called Faustus. Some research pointed to the more Germanic history of the later medieval figure and the name Faust meaning 'fist', but

Faustus in Latin means favoured or lucky. As the now redacted story goes, Vortigen's son was the product of an incestual union and marriage with his own daughter. However, he was fostered to Saint Germanus and led a religious life, although interestingly, he maintained a semi-Pelagian position in the face of the emerging orthodoxy of the Church.

Pelagius, and his views, to me characterises much of the Celtic Church's position, in that spiritual realisation is considered to be available to the endeavours of the individual without recourse to the Church and/or through the figure of Jesus. At least that is my naïve perspective, and it also closely allies with the Jungian psychological idea of individuation. This position is one that foreshadows much of the later Faust legends, as well as the spiritual position of the esoteric Grail legends. Is Vortigern's son and grandson Faustus, even with his odd and probably misinterpreted birth history, in fact Merlin? Is there something here about his continued presence in the Doctor Faustus figure of a millennium later as well as the Grail legends?

Then I turned briefly to Arthur's creation and the remarkable similarities to Vortigern's more notable son, Vortimer, and my head span. I am left with the feeling that Vortigern's story is far more pivotal than has hitherto been considered. At a historical level, I would get utterly lost in trying to put the pieces together. This is at a time when history merges indistinguishably into myth and spirituality; somehow they must be read together and not as separate streams or disciplines.

Yet the Pelagian position seems to me to also inform the Grail legends, at least until they fell into the Church's hands. I started to also glean something distinctly Gnostic in the Faust figure. I also started to intuitively understand why Merlin is an essential figure to these legends, sometimes directly and sometimes via the Arthurian pathway.

Then a final insight loomed. In the Original Dream, the Grail is the dominant feature of the first part, whilst Merlin figures more in the second. Or am I right? Is the jar and the vice a reference more to Faust as magician rather than Merlin? I shied away from this, conditioned as I am to see Faust in some sort of dominating masculine figure with dark connotations in the modern landscape. But is this a splitting of the archetypal magician into good (Merlin) and bad (Faust) also a modern tendency? Does my discovery of Faustus as Vortigern's son and his indirect proximity to Merlin and some potential reconciliation? Does my lingering disquiet about Arthur's conception find a place here? Is Goethe's Faust an attempt to such, with the restoration of the 'eternal feminine'? Is this a potential task for me, as an extension of this work?...

But enough; maybe I have just set out my next writing task, and these insights are not for this work (although they do show the creative process does not cease at the end of the final chapter). My subjectivity was leeching into the relative objectivity of my researches and the disciplines I was exploring. I would want to take this all further, and that is my quest and maybe for some as yet to be defined creative future. Instead, I would round off this work by returning to the positions on which it was written and rests; the above illustrates how the loose ends continue to weave their magic and direct me forward. As Tolkien said: "The road goes ever on."

I now have a different perspective of dualism and the opposites. Relatively, I see this as a way of looking at the world, along with other cognitive functions like causality, quantification and reductionism. When restricted to the mind as the self in the world, they assume a balance, an equality; or at least, that's how we are taught to see them in such a dualistic manner.

After over half a century of training, qualification and practice in the fields of physiological sciences, medicine, psychiatry, depth psychology and comparative religion, supported by an extensive exploration of associated disciplines, I now take a primarily intrapsychic or subjective view of existence that includes an extrapsychic, dualistic and objective worldview, yet also extends far beyond it: It transcends such a primarily and exclusively objective worldview, infinitely and eternally. The mind includes and extends beyond the body, to soul and spirit, yet is included within this greater and increasingly ethereal state of being and experience: The subjective includes the objective, as forgetting does with remembering, yet the former not only includes but also transcends the latter, here and with all such opposites.

The marginal and mirrored borderland between these states of being, such as the objective and subjective, is the domain of the mystic and the magician. The latter is an active equivalent of the more passive former; he or she seeks to work with this greater reality and, at times, bring it into the present and the world. Various attributes and values mark this perspective; prophecy, ecstasy, creativity and healing are amongst them. These values are accessed not through rationality, but the emotional and feeling dimensions of ourselves, encompassing the imagination and including the greater intellect of the abstract and ideas. They are, or have the initial appearance of being irrational and feminine, yet even these apparent gender opposites are transcended the deeper the journey into the infinite and eternal. Here endeth the lesson.

But, in the words of Blake, it outlines a system I have created, as reflected in the idiosyncratic and soulful journeys of many other travellers. The above is merely a summary, relatively fluid and always incomplete, but is portrayed in the pages that precede it. Using this lens – or mirror – is my way of summarising how I see Merlin and The Grail.

In one respect, this whole work could be seen as an *amplification*; in that I have taken material from my personal life and experience, and embellished it with content drawn from collective areas as diverse as myth, the history of others, real and imagined, and culture generally. In that process, this account has expanded and endorsed my own individuation process; it has been a successful (ad)venture. The extension of this process is that I have made such mythic, historical and cultural material relevant to our time. In so doing, I have not exhausted the possibilities, but tried to keep them relevant to my personal narrative. Further extensions would pass more into research, academic and intellectual channels that may not be commensurate with my story.

A further endorsement of at least Jungian principles is that I have used dreams as the mainstay of this process, as well as other material that extends from them, such as personal memories and insights. In so doing, I believe I have found and elaborated a kind of psychic map for my life's journey based on my personal story and the various extensions that is compatible with the concept of individuation, destiny or *wyrd*. It further provides a context of meaning and direction. However, there are various significant areas in which I differ from Jung in the account, which I trust are apparent, but will further elucidate here.

The word *Psyche* is thrown around with abandon. It is a Greek word and literally means *Soul*, but has come in modernity to apply more to the non-physical aspects of our daily existence and, in popular usage, to be seen as synonymous with *Mind*. To tease these conceptual issues out further, I would like to return to the dyads, where I have chosen to approximating apparent opposites with a colon.

Starting with body:mind, which seems straightforward enough where these opposing forces are seen as somehow equal in a qualitative way, as just indicated: Which is why psyche is probably a better term, but now renders the colonic dyad imbalanced, as it appears far greater, more comprehensive and less deniable than body; it is also immaterial, and what are the limits here… indeed, are there any? Has the objective:subjective dyad collapsed too, and do we have to see *subjective* as something far greater as I have already indicated that I do? This is what I am proposing here with considering my personal story to have a psychic relevance that is also transpersonal, collective or spiritual. In fact, all our stories are based on such a psychic bedrock that transcends the one of physical genetics yet also includes it.

There is much more that can be explored in this domain; I have already referenced modern physics as one way. A way I did this was to get out of the straitjacket of my materialistic and scientific thinking, reinforced as it was by medical education, by exploring how the Anglo-Saxons viewed the psyche. What I found was a mythic worldview that mapped quite well onto our current understanding of the brain's physiology, explaining anomalies in a way that my scientific training did and could not. This started to alert me to the limits of our modern scientific worldview, ultimately to marginalise it in ways that I have done frequently in this account.

In brief, my conclusion is that the present era is by no way as progressive or advanced as we would like to think, except in the material, technological and scientific areas, which it has then hypostasised as a concrete and absolute view of existence. I have eschewed this, reversed my lens, and come to see that the mythic, historical (the authentic one and not simply our regressive view of it) and cultural as streams in which the present and my personal existence are embedded. I have given various maps of this throughout the account.

Merlin was specifically created by Geoffrey of Monmouth in the twelfth century. This was a literary and creative act that was grafted onto myth, legend and history in a manner common to the times. The imperative, reasons and intent of this act can only be partially assessed, as I have done here. But the issue is that, once created, he developed an existence that further attracted – or was designed to attract – deeper mythic and spiritual forces. Of relevance to modernity is the significance of the magus or magician, the connection to culture, heritage and a spirituality in danger of being obscured and lost, to act as a prophetic force into the future.

Although a Merlin of whatever name always existed deep in the archetypal imagination, once created he could not be 'unseen' from the manuscripts in which he appeared. As the legends unfolded and the Grail emerged into literature, there were various ways he was dealt with and included in the ongoing cultural trends, most specifically the Church. He was not always to the ecclesiastical liking, but could not now be excluded; although attempts have been made, as with his incarceration. The remembrance of Celtic spirituality and such a figure, who could both compete with Jesus and raise the spectre of Woden, was awkward. Killing two birds with one stone and also dealing with the feminine in a distinctly misogynist manner was also a method of the Church. But Merlin would not be so easily dismissed, as modernity has shown us. He has also not been created; he has always existed. The Arthurian and Grail legends add another layer to Merlin's story, although his presence absents itself at differing points in these stories, and for differing reasons. A revelation to me is how deeply embedded in the Grail he is or has become, even to a profound resonance with Parzival himself.

Of all the themes that have been explored in the Grail legends, the one that intrigues and seems to be most relevant to modernity is that of the feminine. Going back to the dyad, it is tempting to see masculine:feminine as some sort of equivalence. But rather like body:mind, I have come to wonder from the psychic perspective whether the feminine is qualitatively different and more related to terms like 'soul' and even the modern 'unconscious'. I wonder about the relative disconnection between the masculine and feminine portrayed in the myths, questioning if this is reflected elsewhere, even in the structure of our central nervous system. I see the masculine to somehow have emerged – in both a psychic and evolutionary manner – from the feminine, but also to have usurped and diminished her in the process, with all sorts of levels of violation and inevitable consequences, some of which blight us in the modern era.

I suspect there is much in the Grail corpus that tells of this in sexual and violent terms: Who carried the power and magic, I wonder? It seems to me that much of the Grail material is an attempt to restore this balance, such that the trauma and wounding does not continue to afflict us with various wasteland representations and becomes an agent of healing. This is apparent in our era with the continued disempowerment of the feminine; exemplified in women the world over; the ongoing influence and actions of institutions (most notably the Church in our culture); in matters of gender and sexuality; the wasteland represented in climate change, extreme poverty and malnutrition, and our lack of care for the environment. Maybe this is the secret of the Grail.

Although extending from the above and hinted at, the deeper issue of death and such questions as the afterlife haunt this narrative. Maybe this is where my pen will pass to these realms and the questions they arise. But it is time to rest this pen. There is much more than could be said, and this is an inquiry that will continue for me.

The More Poetic Epilogue

I would like to have thought that this account would bring some sense of resolution to the haunting dream that began my journey, at least in a conscious manner. Because this journey was already being undertaken prior; I had just not realised it, or I had finally chosen to take the reins. Yet even that is relative, a delusion maybe, that with my becoming conscious of the process that I then have some sort of control over it. Patently, I do not; in fact, the opposite, as any with a mystical tendency would be inclined to agree with. Yet I have chosen to cooperate with the process and participate in its evolution, under the impression that somehow such awareness makes a difference: Maybe it does not, but is there a choice? Also, I have no conscious resolution; the process simply deepens. The dream, and the others revealed here, have given up more of their secrets, but the haunting feeling is that there is more to come.

Merlin is some kind of Doppelgänger I suspect, who haunts me and reveals more of himself – myself – to me. He sits on the margins, the liminal space that is reflected and somewhat trivialised in the word 'subliminal'. From there he mirrors myself. He did this for Geoffrey and has, and will continue to do, for countless others. In my journey he takes me past my upbringing and its Christian accretions, in so doing relativises this story and its characters, establishing one that is more familiar to my landscape, outer and inner. From there, he led me to The Grail.

Like the Arthurian knights and the King himself, the trials and traumas of my life provided an initiatory challenge with Merlin as a guide. The fantastic imaginations of this journey are my contribution to healing the landscape, the wasteland. It's wounded feminine nature has revealed herself through portals of a psychic nature; the discovery of a core that lies beyond not only my story, but the one we all are given. And it was not just a question of rescuing her; she also rescued me. But I had to face all the wounding of my life that mirrored what had – and still has – occurred to her. That took me beyond.

The Grail was revealed to me through her agency, presenting me with tasks to undertake. Now in the latter time of my life, these have been undertaken; the hallows are revealed. I would like to think the journey ends here, and that I can bask in whatever healing and achievements that have occurred, but I know this not to be the case, there is more to come; isn't there always? For that is the nature of this life for me; I may have cycled to the beginning and a closure of sorts, but it is relative. There is more to be done; I can feel it, and Merlin so advises.

Such is the nature of The Grail.

Postscript

It is now clear to me why I have identified so strongly with Merlin and why he remains embedded in the Grail legends, even the ones of a fundamentally Christian disposition. Merlin is essential to the process, as the magician who leads into the territory of the Grail. Without such an identification, I would have missed the entrance, the portal; even though this is heavily disguised by negative aspects of the feminine as a form of magical censorship. There are two significant themes that this personal Grail exploration has revealed to me, beyond the central one about the level of the Psyche that has talked to and guided me, and how with dreams and their exploration have proved fundamental to this process. The first theme follows this central one, in that individuation into the spiritual realms is a fundamental to achieving the Grail, and that this idiosyncratic journey would attract the accusation of heresy and more in times past. However, with the lessening of the Church's repressive yoke, we live in times where this approach can be made more public, although we still need to be wary of the subtly of modern censorship in these realms. The second is that the negativity of the feminine that Merlin has been weighed down with has paradoxically revealed its opposite; it is through this portal into the realm of the feminine that the Grail is revealed. Healing is revealed as a complex of magic and individuation that reveals our personal destiny and acceptance of the wisdom that suffering contains.

Be the Grail a chalice containing blood, a cauldron of death and rebirth, or the alchemist's stone, matters not. It is ethereal, and would cloak itself in the image of and for the beholder, myself included. I choose to see it in the broader context of the hallows, themselves held in the feminine, with the stone or jewel as the central feature, as in my Original Dream.

Bibliography

NB: The full academic detail, including publisher and date, is not given here; this is easily found with modern technology and may include more current editions.

It is also necessarily brief and not intended to be exhaustive, instead it reflects my personal library in the foregoing inquiry. Any title may open an idiosyncratic inquiry that would probably include a more exhaustive bibliography.

The works outlined are the ones most emotionally significant to me; relevant others may be hinted at in the text of this account.

Merlin
Goodrich, Norma *Merlin*
Knight, Stephen *Merlin: Knowledge and Power Through the Ages*
Lawrence-Mathers, *The True History of Merlin the Magician*
Markale, Jean *Merlin*
Matthews, John *Merlin: Shaman, Prophet, Magician*
Stewart, RJ *The Prophetic Vision of Merlin* & *The Mystic Life of Merlin*
Stewart, RJ & Matthews, John (Ed.) *Merlin Through the Ages*
Tolstoy, Nikolai *The Quest for Merlin*

The Grail
Barber, Richard *The Holy Grail: Imagination and Belief*
Campbell, Joseph *Romance of The Grail*
Jung, Emma & von Franz, Marie-Louise *The Grail Legend*
Knight, Gareth *Merlin and the Grail Tradition*
Loomis, Roger Sherman *The Grail: From Celtic Myth to Christian Symbol*

Markale, Jean *The Grail*

Matthews, John *The Grail: A Secret History*

Matthews, John (Ed.) *At the Table of The Grail*

Weston, Jessie L. *From Ritual to Romance*

Wood, Juliette *The Holy Grail: History & Legend*

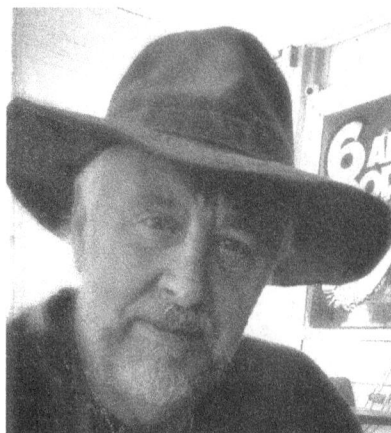

About the Author

My work is with the recovery and reinstatement of the soul, individually and within our modern culture.

By my degrees, qualifications and experience, I am an Oxford and London-trained physiologist and medical doctor; by training and former practice a Jungian analyst; by initiation a Druid and shamanic healer; by decree an ordained priest and an elder in my tradition, and by disposition an alchemist, poet and wordsmith.

My former work as a general practitioner, holistic physician, and medical psychotherapist has been a preparation for this present path.

I am called to wrest from obscurity the ground between a dying religion, and a soul-less science....

Volumes of knowledge and experience to be shared and dispensed to those who ask, and would listen.

An alchemist's robe I wrap around an ageing frame, a magical staff to feel my way, my heart beating to an ancient tune. A poetic sensibility is my torch.

A call to healing, vision and re-enchantment, a social cohesion of like-minded souls, and a community to lead us through the darkest of times.

My heritage is in the northern spiritual traditions, specifically druidry, shamanism, and alchemy.

I bring these into modernity through the agencies and disciplines of medicine, depth psychology, and magic.

My landscape is now Australia; working with people and culture to forge a new identity and direction; clarifying meaning and purpose; grounded in ritual and ceremony, and the offerings that unfold; a direction encapsulated in the beating heart.